Basic Statistics for
Health Science Students

A Series of Books in Psychology

Editors:
Jonathan Freedman
Gardner Lindzey
Richard F. Thompson

Basic Statistics for Health Science Students

David S. Phillips

University of Oregon Medical School

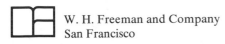

W. H. Freeman and Company
San Francisco

Library of Congress Cataloging in Publication Data

Phillips, David S
  Basic statistics for health science students.

  (A Series of books in psychology)
  Includes index.
  1.   Medical statistics.   I.   Title.
  [DNLM: 1.   Statistics.   2.   Biometry.   HA29 P558b]
  RA409.P495   519'.02'461   77–13865
  ISBN 0–7167–0051–4
  ISBN 0–7167–0050–6 pbk

To Bus, Ben, Dick, and Harold

Contents

Preface

Individuals in the health sciences who are involved in research, directly or indirectly, have come to realize that it is necessary for them to have some familiarity with statistics. Of course, researchers who are actively collecting data must be able to apply statistics, but those who attempt to keep up with the current scientific literature in their fields need also to understand the uses and misuses of statistical techniques. It is for these individuals that this book has been written. It may be used as a text by the individuals who wish to approach the topic of statistics by themselves but is intended more for use as a course textbook or as a quick reference book for students who have previously taken a course in statistics.

Having served as a statistical consultant to the staff and students of a health sciences center and having taught statistics to dental, medical, nursing, and basic medical science Ph.D. students for several years, I have found a need for a simply written introductory book that covers a wide variety of statistical problems. While there are a number of very good introductory textbooks available, most of these do not deal with the types of problems confronted by the health scientist. Furthermore, the need is for a nontheoretical, cookbook approach. Most of the physicians and nurses who have come to me for statistical help have no more interest in the theory underlying a statistical test than they do in the theory underlying the building of an X-ray machine. Both the X ray and the statistical test are viewed as tools that may be useful in answering a particular question. Typically I am asked, "What formula should I use with these data to answer this question and how do I interpret the results?" Hence, this book attempts to cover, in cookbook fashion, a wide variety of statistical techniques that I have found being used by health professionals. It is assumed only that the reader has some familiarity with high-school level algebra.

The topic of statistics may be divided into two broad areas—descriptive statistics and inferential statistics. The first half of this book deals with descriptive statistics commonly encountered in the health sciences, and the second half covers some inferential statistics.

The goal of descriptive statistics is just that—to describe data. In 1975 there were 3728 physicians licensed to practice medicine in Oregon. This statement tells us the population under study but really does not describe it. Depending upon our interests we could describe this population in a variety of ways: the number of physicians in each specialty, their average age, the percent who are females, the patient/physician ratio, etc. When we have data that we wish to describe we may do this either pictorially (tables and graphs) or numerically (ratio, percents, rates, correlation). Most data can be described in more than one way so that the choice of method is up to the investigator. In making this choice the investigator should choose the method that will most clearly present the point that he or she wishes to make with a particular audience. This is to say that the same data may be presented in different forms for different audiences. A student who has done a thesis project on congenital heart disease would present his or her data one way in a talk for the PTA but in a different way in a paper given at the American Heart Association meeting and perhaps in a third way for the defense of his or her thesis before a group of professors.

Just as the person who is presenting that data must be careful in selecting the form to be used in the presentation, so must the consumer be careful. The speaker or writer is going to use the best means available to make his or her point, and the listener or reader must consider that if the data were presented and/or organized in another fashion they might lend themselves to another interpretation. We are used to being skeptical when we read the used-car ads in the newspaper and see cold remedies advertised on TV, but we need that same skepticism when we are confronted with "scientific" data in lectures and journals.

Most chapters have exercises so the student can test his or her understanding of the material. Answers to the exercises are at the end of the book.

I am grateful to the Literary Executor of the late Sir Ronald A. Fisher, F.R.S., to Dr. Frank Yates, F.R.S., and to Longman Group Ltd., London, for permission to reprint Tables III, IV, and VII from their book *Statistical Tables for Biological, Agricultural and Medical Research* (6th edition, 1970).

I also wish to express my appreciation to the Biometrika Trustees for permission to reprint Tables 1 and 18 from E. S. Pearson and H. O. Hartley's *Biometrika Tables for Statisticians, Vol. I,* 3rd edition; to the Institute of Educational Research at Indiana University for permission to reproduce the materials in Appendix E; to the Institute for Mathematical Statistics for permission to reprint the material in Appendix F; to Lederle Laboratories, a division of American Cyanamid Company, for permission to reproduce the material found in Appendix G; and to the American Statistical Association for permission to use the material composing Appendix I and Appendix J.

September 1977   *David S. Phillips*
Portland, Oregon

Basic Statistics for
Health Science Students

Chapter 1
Tables and Graphs

In this chapter we will consider ways to present data in a tabular or graphic fashion. All kinds of data lend themselves to pictorial presentation, and consequently the variety of forms is limited only by one's imagination. Because of the variety of forms, it is impossible to construct a general set of "rules" to be followed in generating tables and graphs. However, authors should keep in mind that the aim is to summarize data; so the material should be presented in a clear and concise manner.

The best way to evaluate a table or a graph is to ask the question, "Can this table or graph stand alone? Is it clear enough to be self-explanatory?" If you have to refer to the text of a journal article to understand a graph, it is not self-sufficient. The best way to make a table self-sufficient is to label it properly. This labeling begins with the title and is carried on throughout the table. The title should contain information about what kind of data are in the table, when the data was collected, where it was collected and who was involved. "Immature births by county of residence, Washington, 1977" tells us exactly what we will find in the accompanying table. The headings in a table and the axes on a graph should be appropriately labeled. In any case where the units of measurement are not obvious, they should be indicated.

Tables

Tables have the general form indicated in Table 1.1. Each table is given a number so that it can be referenced, and this number and the title appear above the table. Headings and subheadings should be clearly labeled. If the table is being used in a talk or an article to quickly make a particular point, it should be kept brief. A table composed of eight columns of numbers covering an 8×11 page does not lend itself to a quick conclusion. Large tables of this type are appropriate for reference works or thesis appendixes where the reader may want access to detailed information for further study.

Table 1.1.   *Title: typical table*

Stub	Heading Subheading	Heading Subheading

Graphs

What we have said about tables also applies to graphs: keep them concise, label them appropriately. Graphs are given numbers also and the number of the figure and its title usually appear below the figure. The variable under study is customarily plotted on the horizontal axis of the graph, the **abscissa;** the vertical axis, the **ordinate,** contains enumerative data, such as the number of cases, rate per 10,000, percentage of patients, etc.

Frequency Polygons

Several forms of graphs occur with such frequency that they have been given specific names. Suppose that we are studying a group of pediatric patients with the following ages: 1, 1, 2, 2, 2, 2, 3, 3, 4, 5, 6. We can plot these data by listing the ages on the abscissa and the number of patients on the ordinate. For each age group we count the number of patients and then put a dot on the graph above that age and corresponding to the number of patients in that group. After we have done this for each age group, we join the points with a line and we extend this line down to the abscissa at each end to keep the graph from hanging in mid-air. This type of graph is called a **frequency polygon.**

Some individuals prefer to use relative frequencies or percentages on the ordinate when plotting data of this nature. As can be seen from comparing the three graphs in Figure 1.1, the overall shape of the figure remains the same regardless of which of these is used on the ordinate. Relative frequencies or percentages may be especially useful when the intent is to compare two or more sets of scores. However, caution should be used when interpreting such data if the numbers of observations are small.

Histograms

If we use the same graph but erect a column proportional to the number of cases at that age at each point on the abscissa, we will produce Figure 1.2, which is a **histogram.** Frequency polygons and histograms can be used to present the same data; so the choice is up to the personal preference of the author. If several sets of data are to be presented simultaneously, this may be done with a frequency polygon. Histograms are usually limited to two sets of data on one figure. As with frequency polygons, histograms may have percentages or relative frequencies plotted on their ordinates.

Ogives

An **ogive** or cumulative percentage curve is generated if we plot the cumulated percent on the ordinate and the age on the abscissa. By picking an age on the abscissa, reading up to the curve and over to the ordinate, we can determine what percent of our patients are below a particular age. For example, from Figure 1.3 we see that 90.9% of our pediatric patients are 5 years of age or younger.

Bar Graphs

Suppose that we are studying the types of accidental deaths occurring in Lincoln County during 1972 and we find the following data: home 4, auto 6, public 5, and occupational 3. We can graph these data by listing the cause of

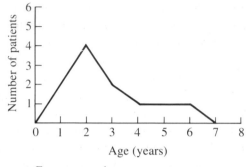

Frequency polygon

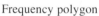

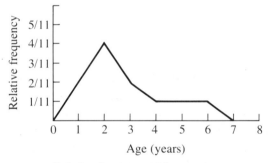

Relative frequency polygon

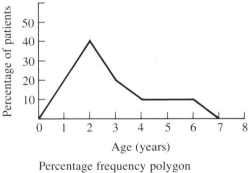

Percentage frequency polygon

Figure 1.1. *Age distribution of pediatric patients in study X, 1976*

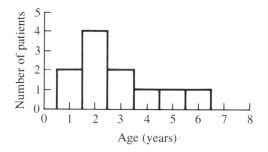

Figure 1.2.   *Histogram of age of pediatric patients in study X, 1976*

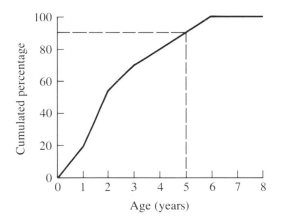

Figure 1.3.   *Ogive of age of pediatric patients in study X, 1976*

death on the abscissa, the number of deaths on the ordinate, and erecting a column proportional to the number of cases of each. This is a **bar graph.** The bar graph (Figure 1.4) and the histogram (Figure 1.2) look very similar, but they are for different types of data. The data plotted on the abscissa of a histogram are assumed to have an underlying continuum and thus can be ordered, that is, age 3 comes before age 4 but after age 2. The data on the abscissa of a bar graph do not have an underlying continuum, and thus order is not important. Deaths from autos could have been plotted first rather than deaths in the home.

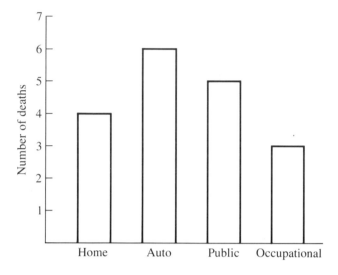

Figure 1.4.   *Bar graph of causes of accidental deaths, Lincoln County, 1972*

Pie Graphs

Another way to present the data in Figure 1.4 pictorially would be to use a **pie diagram.** Here the number of deaths from each cause is converted to a percentage of the total deaths and plotted as a proportional part of a circle or pie as in Figure 1.5.

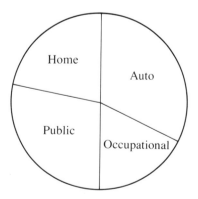

Figure 1.5.   *Pie graph of accidental deaths, Lincoln County, 1972*

Shapes of Distributions

Certain terms are commonly used to describe the shapes of distributions as they deviate from "normal." We will define a "normal distribution" more rigorously in a later chapter, but for now this term is used to refer to a symmetrical, bell-shaped distribution such as Figure 1.6.

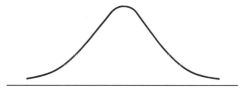

Figure 1.6.   *Normal distribution*

Skewness

If most of the cases pile up at one end of the distribution so that it is no longer symmetrical, we say that the distribution is **skewed.** The tail of the distribution (the end with the smaller number of cases) determines the type of skewness. If the tail is on the left-hand side of the figure, the distribution is negatively skewed (Figure 1.7); if the tail is on the right, it is positively skewed (Figure 1.8).

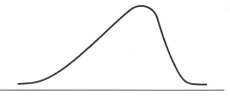

Figure 1.7.   *Negatively skewed distribution*

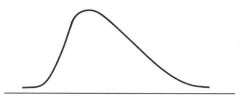

Figure 1.8.   *Positively skewed distribution*

Kurtosis

Skewness tells us something about the symmetry of the distribution. A distribution can be symmetrical and still not be normal. If we grabbed the peak of a normal distribution and either pulled it straight up or pushed it straight down, it would still be symmetrical but it would not be normal. The term **kurtosis** is used to refer to the peakedness of a distribution. A distribution that is flatter than normal is referred to as **platykurtic** (Figure 1.9). A distribution that is more peaked than normal is called **leptokurtic,** while a normal distribution is referred to as **mesokurtic.**

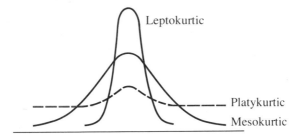

Figure 1.9.   *Types of curves*

Warning

When you are confronted with a table or graph you should ask yourself, "If these data were presented in another way, would they imply another conclusion?" When we see a commercial on TV or an ad in a newspaper we know that someone is trying to sell us something; so we tend to view the material somewhat skeptically. Unfortunately we too often accept articles in scientific journals as proven fact when we should view them skeptically also. The author of a journal article is trying to sell us something too, for instance, that treatment A is superior to treatment B. Study the tables and graphs carefully and do not settle for a first impression.

If we make a frequency polygon of the marriage rate in Oregon for the years 1968–1974, we may vary the overall impression conveyed by the figure by varying the ordinate. Figure 1.10 shows a frequency polygon of these data ranging from a rate of 7.9/1000 in 1968 to 8.8/1000 in 1974. Figure 1.11 is

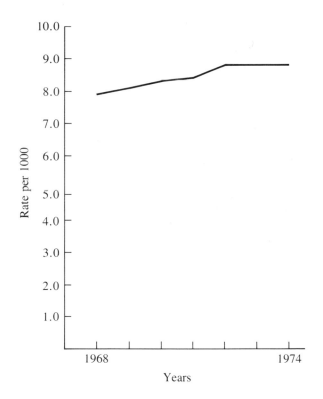

Figure 1.10.   *Marriages in Oregon, 1968–1974*

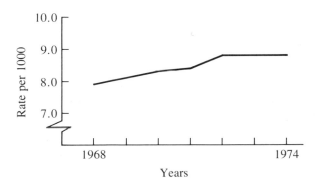

Figure 1.11.   *Marriages in Oregon, 1968–1974*

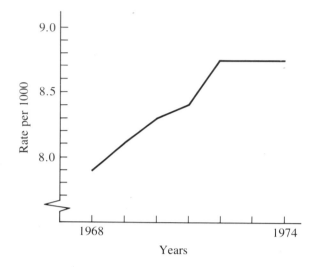

Figure 1.12.   *Marriages in Oregon, 1968–1974*

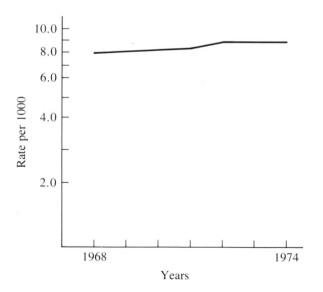

Figure 1.13.   *Marriages in Oregon, 1968–1974*

based on the same data but as it might appear after a journal editor cropped the ordinate to save space. Figures 1.12 and 1.13 also represent the same data, but here the scale on the ordinate has been expanded in 1.12 and reduced in 1.13 by converting to logs. The same data are presented in each of these graphs but the impression conveyed is very different.

Exercise 1

Below are the personal data on 40 cases of rubella.

Patient #	Age	Sex	Race	Duration of Malaise (days)
1	5	M	C	4
2	6	M	B	5
3	8	F	C	1
4	5	M	C	5
5	3	M	B	3
6	6	M	C	4
7	4	F	C	7
8	7	F	C	4
9	5	M	I	6
10	8	F	C	5
11	6	M	B	4
12	5	F	C	3
13	10	F	C	5
14	4	M	B	8
15	6	M	B	2
16	9	M	C	4
17	4	M	B	5
18	6	F	I	4
19	5	M	B	3
20	8	F	C	6
21	5	M	C	5
22	4	M	B	3
23	7	F	C	4
24	7	M	B	7
25	5	M	C	2
26	6	M	C	3

Patient #	Age	Sex	Race	Duration of Malaise (days)
27	4	F	I	5
28	9	M	B	4
29	5	M	C	4
30	5	M	B	4
31	7	M	B	4
32	4	M	C	5
33	8	F	C	4
34	5	F	B	5
35	6	M	I	5
36	4	F	C	3
37	7	F	B	4
38	6	M	B	4
39	5	M	I	3
40	6	F	C*	4

*B = Black, C = Caucasian, I = Indian

Using these data make, title, and label the following figures:

1. a frequency polygon and a relative frequency polygon of the age of the patients,
2. a bar graph of the sex of the patients,
3. a pie graph of the race of the patients, and
4. an ogive for the duration of the malaise.

Chapter 2
Ratios, Proportions, Percentages, and Rates

When we wish to compare two sets of numbers we may make a comparison in terms of their absolute values or in terms of their relative values. Suppose that we wish to compare the population growth in Benton County and Multnomah County from 1960 to 1970:

	1960	1970
Benton County	39,165	53,776
Multnomah County	522,813	556,667

Benton County had an increase in population of 14,611 over this ten-year period while Multnomah County gained 33,853. Comparing these absolute values, Multnomah County had over twice the population gain experienced by Benton County. However, Benton County gained 14,611 individuals from a starting population of 39,165, so that it experienced a 37% increase in its population while Multnomah County gained 33,853 from 522,813, or only a 6% rise. Here we are comparing the increase in population relative to the starting population of each county, and with this type of comparison we see that Benton County has experienced the larger population increase.

Absolute and relative comparisons may lead to the same or to different conclusions, as in the example above. The point to remember is that they are different kinds of comparisons representing different ideas. The statistics that we will consider in this chapter—ratios, proportions, percentages and rates—are all relative measurements.

Ratios

Ratios are the simplest form of relative measurement. To form a ratio we divide the population under consideration into two parts, A and B, and form a fraction of these two numbers. The ratio is expressed as so many cases of A to one case of B:

$$\text{Ratio} = A/B$$

The only requirements are that the same units of measurement be used in both the numerator and the denominator and that the data be collected over the same time period. For example, suppose that we wish to contrast the number of legitimate births to the number of illegitimate births in Oregon during 1973. We find that there were 2,599 illegitimate births and 28,303 legitimate births during that year in Oregon. The ratio of legitimate to illegitimate births would be $28,303/2,599 = 10.9$ to 1. We have split the population of live births into two parts (legitimate and illegitimate); the same unit of measurement has been used in the numerator and the denominator (a live birth); and the data in the numerator and the denominator have been collected over the same period of time (1973).

Proportions

We have seen that ratios are formed by dividing the population into two parts, A and B, and then putting one part over the other. Proportions and percentages are formed by dividing the population into two parts and then putting one part over the total population:

$$\text{Proportion of } A = \frac{A}{A + B}$$

Continuing with the example we used above, the proportion of illegitimate births in Oregon during 1973 would be:

$$\frac{2,599}{2,599 + 28,303} = 0.084$$

Percentages

If we multiply a proportion by 100, we have a percentage. Thus the percentage of illegitimate births in Oregon during 1973 was:

$$\frac{2,599}{2,599 + 28,303} \times 100 = 8.4\%$$

Like ratios, proportions and percentages require that the numerator and the denominator be measured in the same units of measurement and over the same period of time.

Rates

Rates differ from ratios, proportions, and percentages in that while their numerators are accumulated over a period of time (usually a year), their denominators are static figures estimating the population at one point in time. A rate may be defined as:

$$\text{Rate of } X = \frac{\text{Number of cases of } X}{\text{Population at risk to } X} \times \text{base}$$

The numerator is a tabulation of the number of cases of the disease that we have recorded during a specific time interval; the denominator is an estimate of the population at risk of having that disease during that time period; and the base is 10 raised to a power sufficient to report the rate in whole numbers.

In 1973 the State of Oregon recorded 655 deaths from autos, and the population of the state was estimated to be 2,224,900 on July 1, 1973. The auto mortality rate for Oregon during 1973 would be:

$$\frac{655}{2,224,900} = 0.000294$$

but since it is hard for some of us to visualize a 0.000294th of a person, we choose a base of 10,000. Thus:

$$\text{Auto mortality rate, Oregon, 1973} = \frac{655}{2,224,900} \times 10,000 = 2.94/10,000$$

Crude Rates

It should be noted that while the denominator of a rate is always defined as the "population at risk" it may not always be convenient or possible to actually specify these individuals. For example, most birth rates use as their denominators the total population of the area under study. The risk to women under 10 or over 50 years of age is minimal while the risk to males is nonexistent. In this case it is inconvenient to determine what part of the total population is female and of child-bearing age.

If we compute our rate using all the cases of X in the numerator and the total population at risk in the denominator, this is referred to as a crude rate. Examples of crude rates would be:

$$\text{Crude birth rate of U.S., 1976} = \frac{\text{No. live births in U.S., 1976}}{\text{Population of U.S., 7/1/76}} \times 10,000$$

Crude mortality rate of California, 1976

$$= \frac{\text{No. deaths in Calif., 1976}}{\text{Population of Calif., 7/1/76}} \times 10,000$$

Two rates that are frequently encountered, and confused, are prevalence rates and incidence rates. With **incidence rates** we are concerned with the number of new cases that occur during a set time period, whereas **prevalence rates** consider the total number of active cases—the new cases plus the already existing cases.

In order to calculate the incidence rate of flu for the month of January, we would divide the number of reported new cases of flu occurring during the month of January by the population at risk of having flu as of January 1. To compute the prevalence rate of flu for January we would use as our numerator all the newly reported cases of flu during January plus all the cases that had been reported before January 1 but were still active as of that date. This would be an interval prevalence rate. Point prevalence rates may also be computed if we consider the rate for a specific day. The prevalence rate for January 10 would be found by dividing all the active cases of flu on January 10 (old plus new) by the population at risk of having flu as of January 10. This would be a point prevalence rate.

Specific Rates

If the numerator and/or denominator of a crude rate is fractionated, then we have a **specific rate.** For instance, we can take the total number of deaths occurring in California during 1976 and classify these according to cause:

cancer, heart disease, auto, etc. If we took the total population of the state of California and used each of these numbers as numerators we could generate "cause specific mortality rates" for cancer, heart disease, etc., for the state of California. If we break the total population of the state down into ten-year age brackets—0–9, 10–19, etc.—we could determine the number of deaths in each of these age categories and compute "age specific mortality rate":

Age specific mortality rate for 20–29-year-olds, California, 1975

$$= \frac{\text{No. deaths in 20–29 ages}}{\text{Population of 20–29-year-olds, Calif., 1975}} \times 1000$$

If we have two areas and we wish to compare these two areas, then crude rates will give us a realistic comparison only if the two areas are alike with regard to any and all variables that might effect the rates. If this is not the case, then we are not comparing like situations with each other. Consider an extreme example:

Town A is a suburban community with a population of 10,000. The average household is composed of a couple in their mid-twenties with two children. Town B is a retirement community with a population of 10,000. The average household is composed of a couple in their sixties with no children living at home.

If you were told what the crude birth rate and the crude mortality rate were for Town A and for Town B and that was the only information that you were given about these two towns, you would probably wonder what the problem was in Town B since it has a zero birth rate and a high mortality rate. The two towns have different age distributions, and since age influences birth rates and mortality rates, it does not make sense to compare the crude rates in this case. Once we know that Town B is a retirement center we are not surprised by the birth rate or mortality rate. Specific rates allow us to break the total population down into units that are similar to each other so that we can compare like units in the two populations.

Let us consider another example, this time from the real world. In Oregon during 1960 there were 16,779 deaths from all causes and the population was estimated as 1,768,400; during 1970 in Oregon there were 19,520 and an estimated population of 2,091,400.

$$\text{Crude mortality rate, Oregon, 1960} = \frac{16,779}{1,768,400} \times 10,000 = 94.8/10,000$$

$$\text{Crude mortality rate, Oregon, 1970} = \frac{19,520}{2,091,400} \times 10,000 = 93.3/10,000$$

Table 2.1.   *Mortality by age and sex, Oregon, 1960*

Age	Male Population	Number of Deaths	Rate per 10,000	Female Population	Number of Deaths	Rate per 10,000
0–4	94,200	604	64.1	91,200	446	48.9
5–14	183,200	98	5.3	176,600	55	3.1
15–24	110,100	175	15.9	116,500	68	5.8
25–34	99,400	180	18.1	104,100	93	8.9
35–44	115,600	409	35.4	119,800	242	20.2
45–54	108,700	980	90.2	105,100	446	42.4
55–64	80,700	1722	213.4	79,600	822	103.3
65–74	59,000	2627	445.3	61,500	1557	253.2
75+	28,900	3241	1121.5	34,200	3014	881.3
	879,800	10,036	114.0	888,600	6743	75.9

Crude Mortality Rate, Oregon, 1960: 94.9 per 10,000
Source: Oregon State Health Division, *Vital Statistics Annual Report, 1960.*

We see that the crude rate has decreased 1.5/10,000 over this ten-year in-terval. The question that we have to ask ourselves is: "Are these two popula-tions alike with regard to any variable that might influence the rates?" We have already pointed out that age is one variable that should be considered in mortality rates; sex is another. Table 2.1 gives the population of Oregon in 1960 by age and sex. Table 2.2 has the same information for 1970. If we look at the data for females, we see that the sex specific mortality rate for females is:

Sex specific mortality rate, females, Oregon, 1960

$$= \frac{6{,}743}{888{,}600} \times 10{,}000 = 75.9/10{,}000$$

Sex specific mortality rate, females, Oregon, 1970

$$= \frac{8{,}188}{1{,}067{,}500} \times 10{,}000 = 76.7/10{,}000$$

Thus the rate for females has gone up over this ten-year period. However if we look at the age distribution of the females in 1960 and 1970, we see that a larger percentage of the 1970 population is 75 years of age or older. Thus we fractionate the female part of the population even further into ten-year age categories and compute age specific rates for females for 1960 and 1970. Comparing these we see that of the nine age categories the 1970 rate exceeds

Table 2.2.   *Mortality by age and sex, Oregon, 1970*

Age	Male Popualtion	Number of Deaths	Rate per 10,000	Female Population	Number of Deaths	Rate per 10,000
0–4	83,800	367	43.8	80,200	308	38.4
5–14	206,900	117	5.7	198,700	57	2.9
15–24	176,500	351	19.9	189,500	141	7.4
25–34	126,600	196	15.5	128,000	110	8.6
35–44	110,500	377	34.1	115,300	203	17.6
45–54	119,000	990	83.2	124,400	537	43.2
55–64	100,400	2027	201.9	104,800	999	95.3
65–74	62,800	2749	437.7	73,100	1647	225.3
75+	37,400	4158	1111.8	53,500	4186	782.4
	1,023,900	11,332	110.6	1,067,500	8188	76.7

Crude Mortality Rate, Oregon, 1970: 93.2 per 10,000
Source: Oregon State Health Division, *Vital Statistics Annual Report, 1970.*

the corresponding 1960 rate only for the 15–24 and 45–54-year-olds. The same procedure has been followed for the data on the male part of the population.

We started by wishing to compare mortality in Oregon during 1960 and 1970, and so we computed two crude rates, one for each year. Next we decided to consider the possible influence of sex in these rates; so we computed four sex specific mortality rates. Finally we broke these down into ten-year age groups and ended up with 36 age-sex specific mortality rates. While these 36 rates are more revealing than the crude rates, we are now in the position of not being able to see the forest for the trees—how can we compare 36 rates and come to some conclusion about mortality in 1960 and 1970? The complicated answer to this simple problem is the use of standardized rates.

Standardized Rates

If we have two sets of specific rates computed using different populations and our goal is to compare the two populations, this can be done using standardized rates. In order to standardize rates the first step is to compute the specific rates on the two populations. We have already done this and they are given in Tables 2.1 and 2.2. The second step is to obtain a standard population. This may be done in several ways, but it is best to use a standard population that has been used before, if an appropriate one can be obtained. We will use the "standard million" used by the U.S. Office of Vital Statistics. This population, broken down by age and sex, is listed in Table 2.3. The third step is to apply the specific rates that were computed in step one to the corresponding part of the standard population to determine the number of cases that would be expected in the standard population if that specific rate held. For example, the rate for 1960, males 0–4 was 64.1 per 10,000, and if this rate held in a population of 40,800 we would expect 262 deaths. Columns 4–8 in Table 2.3 give the expected cases for males and females, 1960 and 1970. The fourth step is to sum up columns 4–8 to determine the total number of cases expected for males and females in 1960 and 1970. Using these sums and the standard population we can compute standardized sex specific rates for the two years:

Standardized sex specific mortality rate, males, Oregon, 1960

$$= \frac{4,678}{515,800} \times 10,000 = 90.7/10,000$$

Standardized sex specific mortality rate, males, Oregon, 1970

$$= \frac{4,479}{515,800} \times 10,000 = 86.8/10,000$$

Standardized sex specific mortality rate, females, Oregon, 1960

$$= \frac{2,508}{484,000} \times 10,000 = 51.8/10,000$$

Standardized sex specific mortality rate, females, Oregon, 1970

$$= \frac{2,277}{484,000} \times 10,000 = 47.0/10,000$$

Note that with the standardized rates, the sex specific rate for females shows a decrease from 1960 to 1970.

We can also combine the data for males and females for each year and compute a standardized mortality rate for each year:

Standardized mortality rate, Oregon, 1960

$$= \frac{7,186}{1,000,000} \times 10,000 = 71.9/10,000$$

Standardized mortality rate, Oregon, 1970

$$= \frac{6,756}{1,000,000} \times 10,000 = 67.6/10,000$$

These two standardized rates have been computed on the same population so that any differences in age or sex distribution have been eliminated. Table 2.4 compares the crude and standardized rates for 1960 and 1970.

Table 2.3.   *Standardization of mortality rates for Oregon, 1960 and 1970*

Age	Standard Population		Deaths Expected in Std. Population 1960		Deaths Expected in Std. Population 1970	
	Males	*Females*	*Males*	*Females*	*Males*	*Females*
0–4	40,800	39,300	262	192	179	151
5–14	86,900	83,400	46	26	50	24
15–24	91,200	90,500	145	52	181	67
25–34	83,000	79,100	150	70	129	68
35–44	71,400	67,800	253	137	243	119
45–54	62,600	55,200	565	234	521	238
55–64	43,600	36,700	930	379	880	350
65–74	25,800	22,600	1149	572	1129	509
75+	10,500	9,600	1178	846	1167	751
	515,800	484,200	4678	2508	4479	2277

Table 2.4.   *Comparison of mortality rates for Oregon, 1960 and 1970*

Types of Mortality Rate	Rates per 10,000	
	1960	1970
Crude	94.8	93.3
Sex specific, female	75.9	76.7
Sex specific, male	114.0	110.6
Age standardized, sex specific, female	51.8	47.0
Age standardized, sex specific, male	90.7	86.8
Standardized for age and sex	71.9	67.6

Life Tables

Life tables are a way of expressing mortality rates for part of or all of a population so that we can estimate what part of the population will be alive at a particular age or what part of the population will die between two specified ages. Life tables are used by insurance companies to determine life expectancies and thus to set premiums. They may also be used to evaluate the long-term effects of various medical treatments.

Suppose that we had 100,000 male infants all born on January 1, 1970, and that we followed these infants until everyone of them had died. Each January 1 we would record how many of our subjects had died during the past year.

To construct a life table we would begin by listing the ages and determining the probability of dying at each age. This is done by dividing the number of deaths that occurred during that year by the number of individuals alive at the start of that year. Using this approach it might be over 100 years before all of our 100,000 subjects had died and we could complete our life table. In order to speed construction up we can use existing mortality rates for our calculations.

We find that the mortality rate for 0–1-year-olds in our state is 148/10,000; for 1–2-year-olds 9/10,000; for 2–3-year-olds 9/10,000; for 3–4-year-olds 8/10,000; 4–5-year-olds 7/10,000; 5–6-year-olds 5/10,000; etc. The probability that an individual will survive a particular age is equal to:

$$\frac{2(\text{that age's mortality rate per person})}{2 + (\text{that age's mortality rate per person})}$$

For age 0–1:

$$\frac{2(.0148)}{2 + .0148} = .0147$$

For age 1–2:

$$\frac{2(.0009)}{2 + .0009} = .0009$$

For age 2–3:

$$\frac{2(.0009)}{2 + .0009} = .0009$$

These values are computed for each age and entered in column #2 of our life table (Table 2.5). If we subtract the probability of dying during the year from 1, we arrive at the probability of an individual surviving that year. For example, the probability that a person who has reached his first birthday will survive till his second birthday is 0.9991 from column #3. If we start with a hypothetical 100,000 individuals at age zero, we can apply our probabilities to this number and determine the number who would be expected to die during each age (column #5) and the number expected to be alive at the beginning of each age (column #4).

Once we have completed columns 1–5 in Table 2.5 we could compute the average life expectancy of those who have reached a particular age. This is done by multiplying the number of people who died at each age by that age plus 0.5 and summing all the values for that age group and those older than

Table 2.5. *Life table*

Age	Probability of Dying During Year	Probability of Surviving the Year	Number Alive at Start of the Year	Number Dying During the Year	Mean Life Expectancy
0	.0147	.9853	100,000	1470	
1	.0009	.9991	98,530	89	
2	.0009	.9991	98,441	89	
3	.0008	.9992	98,352	79	
4	.0007	.9993	98,273	69	
5	.0005	.9995	98,204	49	
6	.0004	.9996	98,155	39	
7	.0003	.9997	98,116	29	
8	.0002	.9998	98,087	20	
.	.	.	98,067	.	
.	.	.	.	.	
.	.	.	.	.	

that age group. This sum is divided by the number of individuals alive at the start of that year. Thus the average life expectancy for all 100,000 individuals would be:

$$[(1470 \times 0.5) + (89 \times 1.5) + (89 \times 2.5) + (79 \times 3.5) + \cdots]/100,000$$

The average life expectancy for those individuals who had reached their third birthday is:

$$[(79 \times 3.5) + (69 \times 4.5) + (49 \times 5.5) + (39 \times 6.5) + \cdots]/98,352$$

Exercise 2

During 1977, 2000 primary cases and 40 secondary cases of "O" virus were reported in the county. The population of the county was 450,000.

1. What is the ratio of primary to secondary cases?
2. What is the proportion of secondary cases?
3. What is the primary attack rate in the county?

Chapter 3

Measures of Central Tendency

Central tendency is a term that statisticians use for "average." When we compute a measure of central tendency we are attempting to describe a set of scores by using one score or number. For instance, if we have a class of 30 students, we could list each person's weight or we could summarize these 30 scores by saying that the average weight for the class was "B."

Consider the five numbers 1, 1, 2, 8, and 64. What is their average? Unfortunately the term "average" is a generic term that includes several different sets of computations. For the five scores above, the following averages may be calculated: mode = 1.0, harmonic mean = 1.89, median = 2.0, geometric mean = 4.0, and arithmetic mean = 15.2—five scores and five different averages! It is for this reason that in scientific writing the term "average" is replaced by the specific type of measure used.

Measures of Central Tendency—Raw Scores

In analyzing data from the health sciences only three of these measures of central tendency are commonly encountered, and we will limit our discussion to these three: the mode, the median, and the mean.

Mode (*Mo*)

The **mode** (*Mo*) is defined as the most frequently occurring score in a set of scores. With regard to the five scores above, the score of 1 occurs twice while all the other scores occur only once; so *Mo* = 1. The mode has the disadvantage of not always being uniquely defined for a given set of scores. The scores 1, 1, 2, 3, and 3 would be bimodal since the score of 1 occurs twice and the score of 3 occurs twice.

Median (*Md*)

The **median** (*Md*) is defined as the middle score in a set of ordered scores. The scores 1, 1, 2, 8, and 64 are already ordered; so *Md* = 2.0. There are two scores smaller than 2 and two scores larger than 2. If we have an even number of scores, then the median is that point half way between the middle two scores after they have been ordered. For example, the median for the set of scores 1, 2, 3, and 4 is *Md* = 2.5.

Mean ($\overline{X}$)

The arithmetic mean ($\overline{X}$), usually referred to simply as the **mean,** is defined as:

$$\overline{X} = \frac{\Sigma X}{N} \qquad (3\text{--}1)$$

In statistical jargon the Greek capital letter sigma (Σ) is used to indicate addition, and X denotes a raw score. The symbol N refers to the number of raw scores; so $\Sigma X/N$ tells us to add up all the raw scores and then divide this total by the number of scores that we have. For our scores of 1, 1, 2, 8, and 64, $\Sigma X = 76$ and there are five scores; so $\overline{X} = 76/5 = 15.2$.

Measures of Central Tendency—Grouped Data

So far we have discussed situations where we had access to the raw scores or all of the data. In situations involving a large number of observations one may not have access to individual raw scores but rather these data may already be summarized or grouped. If we wanted to determine the average birth weight of infants born in Oregon during 1972, the Oregon State Health Division would provide us with Table 3.1 rather than a list of the 32,400 actual birth weights. Let us compute our three averages on these data.

Table 3.1.   *Birth weights in grams of Oregon infants, 1972*

Weight	f	MP	$f(MP)$	$f(MP)^2$
0–500	0	250.5	0	0
501–1000	100	750.5	75,050	56,325,025
1001–1500	200	1250.5	250,100	312,750,050
1501–2000	300	1750.5	525,150	919,275,075
2001–2500	1,200	2250.5	2,700,600	6,077,700,300
2501–3000	5,000	2750.5	13,752,500	37,826,251,250
3001–3500	12,000	3250.5	39,006,000	126,789,003,000
3501–4000	10,000	3750.5	37,505,000	140,662,502,500
4001–4500	3,000	4250.5	12,571,500	54,200,250,750
4501–5000	500	4750.5	2,375,250	11,283,625,125
5001–5500	100	5250.5	525,050	2,756,775,025
	32,400		109,466,200	380,884,458,100

Mode

When considering raw scores we defined the mode as the most frequently occurring score; with grouped data the mode is defined as the midpoint of the interval containing the most scores. The interval 3001–3500 containing 12,000 scores has more scores than any other interval; so its midpoint is the mode, $Mo = 3250.5$ grams.

In working with grouped data we must know how the groups were set up so that we know what the dividing point is between two adjacent groups. In our present example, birth weights were recorded to the nearest gram; so the point dividing two intervals is 0.5, that is, a 3500.4-gram infant would be counted in the 3100–3500 gram group, and one weighing 3500.7 grams would be in the 3501–4000 group. Usually data are grouped to the nearest gram, pound, inch, mm Hg, mg%, etc., but age is a common exception. Age is more commonly recorded in terms of the last birthday so that a person who will be 20 tomorrow is considered to be 19 today even though he is closer to his twentieth birthday. Here the point separating the groups would be 19.99.

Median

The median is the score that divides our set of scores into two equal halves each containing $N/2$ scores in it. In our example we have 32,400 infants; so the point that we are seeking will have $32,400/2 = 16,200$ scores above it and

16,200 scores below it. If we start at the top of the table we see that there are not any infants weighing less than 500 grams. There are 100 infants weighing less than 1000.5 grams, 300 weighing less than 1500.5 grams, 600 weighing less than 2000.5 grams, 1800 weighing less than 2500.5 grams, 6800 weighing less than 3000.5 grams, and 18,800 weighing less than 3500.5 grams. Therefore our 16,200th score is somewhere in the interval 3000.5–3500.5, and we must interpolate to find this point. Starting at the lower limit of this interval (3000.5) we have 6800 infants weighing less than 3000.5 grams, and we need 9400 more infants out of this interval to give us the 16,200th score (16,200 − 6800 = 9400). Now since the total number of infants in the next interval is 12,000 and since the interval is 500 grams wide, we need 9400/12,000s of 500. So the median is:

$$Md = 3000.5 + \frac{9,400}{12,000}(500) = 3000.5 + 391.7 = 3392.2$$

In computing the median we started at the top of Table 3.1 and worked downward. We can also start at the bottom of the table and work upward. If we take this approach, we find that there are 13,600 infants weighing more than 3500.5 grams and that we need 16,200 − 13,600 = 2,600 more scores out of the interval 3000.5 − 3500.5. So:

$$Md = 3500.5 - \frac{2,600}{12,000}(500) = 3500.5 - 108.3 = 3392.2$$

(Note that in this case the median is something less than 3500.5, so that the fraction is subtracted.)

Mean

In computing the mean for a set of raw scores the first step was to sum all the raw scores, but with grouped data we do not have access to the individual raw scores. We know that within each interval there is a certain number of scores, but we can not specify what each individual score is. In this situation the best that we can do is to estimate all the scores in a given interval with the midpoint (MP) of that interval. If we multiply the number of scores in the interval by the midpoint of the interval, we can use this as an estimate of the sum of all the scores in that interval, $f(MP)$. If we do this for each interval and then sum all of these and divide by N, we have computed the mean. In Table 3.1 column #3 lists the midpoints of the intervals and column #4 lists the product of the midpoint of the interval and the number of scores in that interval. Summing column #4 we obtain 109,466,200, and the mean is:

$$\overline{X} = \frac{\Sigma f(MP)}{N} = \frac{109,466,200}{32,400} = 3378.6 \qquad (3-2)$$

Scales of Measurement

We have discussed how to compute the mode, median, and mean for a set of raw scores or for grouped data. Since we have spent the time to consider three different measures of central tendency, you hay have guessed that these measures have different uses. Consider the statement, "The average baby born last week at County Hospital was male, weighing 3490 grams with an Apgar score of eight and a body temperature of 37°C." In this one sentence we have used four measures of central tendency: one mode, one median, and two means. Why? The answer is that we can collect data in different ways and the way in which the data are collected dictates what can be done with them. When we measure or collect data we do this according to certain rules or scales of measurement.

Nominal Scale

The simplest scale of measurement is called a **nominal scale,** and the only restriction is that all of the objects put into one group must have something in common with each other and be different from objects in other groups. When we classify patients by sex this is a nominal scale: one group contains all the females; everyone in this group has something in common; and they are different from individuals put into the male group. Classifying people by blood type (A, B, AB, O) is another example of a nominal scale. Note that if numbers are used with a nominal scale to designate groups—Group #1, Group #2, etc.—these numbers are used as labels only and can not be manipulated mathematically.

When we analyze nominal data we can determine whether we have more males than females or which blood type occurs with the greatest frequency, that is, we can compute a mode. In fact, with nominal scale data, the mode is the only measure of central tendency that we may compute.

Ordinal Scale

Suppose that we retain the idea of grouping from the nominal scale and add the restriction that the variable that we are measuring has an underlying continuum so that we may speak of a person having "more than" or "less than" another person does of the variable in question. This would be an **ordinal scale** or rank order scale of measurement. If we took twenty people with blue eyes and put them into three groups of light blue, blue, or dark blue, this would be an ordinal scale. People put into the blue group have something in common with everyone else in that group and differ from people in the other two groups with regard to the blueness of their eyes. People in the blue group have more blueness than do people in the light blue group and less than do those in the dark blue group. If numbers are used to designate the groups in this instance, they convey the idea of order. Since we can speak of a person possessing more of or less of the trait than does another person, we can order people with regard to the amount of the variable that they possess and then find the middle person, in other words, we can compute a median if we have ordinal scale data.

Interval Scale

The next higher scale of measurement is an **interval scale.** In addition to the criteria of grouping and underlying continuum of the ordinal scale, the interval scale has equal units of measurement. If we inspect a thermometer we see that it is marked off in equal units and the °C and °F scales are interval scales. With equal units of measurement it is permissible to multiply and divide; so we may compute a mean.

Ratio Scale

The last scale of measurement is a **ratio scale.** It requires a true or absolute zero point in addition to grouping, an underlying continuum, and equal units of measurement. By a true zero point we mean that zero on this scale indicates a complete absence of the trait being measured. Height and weight are ratio scales since zero height or weight indicates that the object does not possess these characteristics. Zero on the °F temperature scale does not mean that we do not have any temperature; so this is an interval scale.

To summarize, the first thing that we must consider when computing a measure of central tendency is the scale of measurement used in collecting the data. If the data are nominal, the only measure that we may compute is the mode. If the data are ordinal, we are allowed to compute a mode and a median. If the data are interval or ratio scale, we may compute a mode, a median, or a mean.

Distribution of Scores and Central Tendency

Suppose that we have two groups of patients with mumps. The ages for group #1 are: 3, 4, 4, 5, 5, 5, 6, 6, and 7; and for group #2: 3, 4, 4, 5, 6, 7, 8, 10, and 43. Since age is measured on a ratio scale we may compute all three of our measures of central tendency, and for the two groups these are:

	Mo	Md	$\overline{X}$
Group #1	5	5	5
Group #2	4	6	10

In group #1 all of the averages have the same numerical value: $Mo = Md = \overline{X} = 5$; in group #2 all of the averages are different, ranging from 4 to 10. If we make a histogram of each of the sets of scores, Figure 3.1, we see that they have different distributions.

Group #1 has a symmetrical distribution, and whenever we have a symmetrical distribution all three of our averages will be numerically equal. Group #2 has a skewed distribution rather than a symmetrical one, and hence the averages have different numerical values. In a skewed distribution the mode will be at the highest point on the graph; the mean will fall toward the tail of the distribution; and the median will tend to fall between the mode and the mean. The more the distribution deviates from being symmetrical, in other words, the more skewed it is, the more our three averages will differ from each other numerically.

The point to keep in mind is that the "average" is the one number that is supposed to represent the whole set of scores. If we have a nominal scale variable, the only average that we may compute is a mode so that we are not faced with a choice. If we have ordinal scale data, we are confronted with a choice between the median and the mode. In this case the mode will be the more representative if we have a peaked distribution; otherwise we should choose the median. With interval or ratio scale data we should choose the mean if the distribution is symmetrical; the median if the distribution is skewed; and the mode if the data are peaked.

The choice of the proper measure of central tendency is determined by two things. First, the scale of measurement determines which measures may be computed. Second, the shape of the distribution tells us which is the most representative measure of those that are allowed.

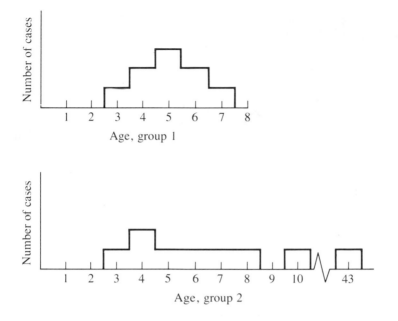

Figure 3.1. *Age distributions of two groups of patients with mumps*

Exercise 3

The incubation period of 50 cases of "O" virus are listed below. Calculate the mode, median, and mean incubation period for this virus. Which of these measures would be the most appropriate for these data? Why?

Incubation period of cases of "O" virus

2	8	6	4	3
4	5	3	3	2
4	5	6	4	3
8	3	7	3	4
5	5	6	2	3
3	4	3	5	2
4	3	2	5	3
6	3	5	4	4
7	9	10	3	3
6	3	2	9	4

Chapter 4

Measures of Variability

When we calculate an average for a set of scores we are describing the center of that set of scores. However, as can be seen in Figure 4.1, we might have several different distributions all with the same center. Therefore, to adequately describe a set of data we need not only a measure of central tendency but also some measure of how the scores are dispersed about that average, a measure of variability.

Measures of Variability—Raw Scores

Range

The simplest measure of variability is the **range.** The range is defined as the difference between the largest and the smallest scores:

$$\text{Range} = \text{Largest score} - \text{Smallest score}$$

Considering the scores 1, 1, 2, 2, 2, 3, 7, and 9, the range is $9 - 1 = 8$. The range has the advantage of being easy to compute, especially if the number

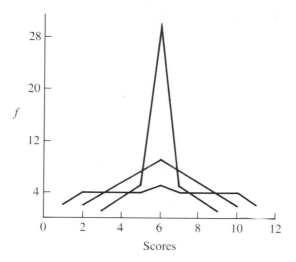

Figure 4.1. *Three distributions having the same mean*

of scores is small or if they have already been arranged in order. However, the range uses only two scores, and these are the two most extreme scores, which tend to be unreliable. Furthermore, it tells us nothing about how the scores are dispersed between these two extremes.

Semi-interquartile Range (Q)

The **semi-interquartile range** (Q) is another measure of variability that is more stable than the range but more time consuming in its computation. Q is defined as half the distance between the first and third quartile:

$$Q = \frac{Q_3 - Q_1}{2} \tag{4–1}$$

The first quartile (Q_1) is that point in the distribution with 25% of the scores below it, and the third quartile (Q_3) is that point with 75% of the scores below it. (Note that Q_2 has 50% of the scores below it and hence is the same as the median.) Consider the scores: 1, 1, 2, 2, 3, 4, 5, and 8.

$Q_1 = 1.5$ (Two out of the eight scores are below this value.)

$Q_3 = 4.5$ (Six out of the eight scores are below this value.)

$Q = \dfrac{4.5 - 1.5}{2} = 1.5$

If we have interval or ratio scale data, we could use an averaging process similar to that used in calculating the mean. If we have a set of scores for which we have computed the mean and we want to describe how the scores vary about this mean, then why not calculate the difference between each score and the mean, sum these, and divide by the number of scores:

$$\frac{\Sigma(X - \overline{X})}{N} \qquad (4-2)$$

If we look at the five scores—1, 2, 3, 4, and 5—we see that their mean is 3.0; so we can subtract this value from each score:

X	$X - \overline{X}$
1	-2
2	-1
3	0
4	1
5	2

$$0 = \Sigma(X - \overline{X})$$

The fact that $\Sigma(X - \overline{X}) = 0$ is not unique for this set of numbers but is true for any set. To circumvent this problem two approaches have been taken historically.

Average Deviation (*AD*)

If we compute the absolute difference between each score and the mean, then we will end up with a positive number that can be divided by N. This is called the **Average deviation** (*AD*):

$$AD = \frac{\Sigma|X - \overline{X}|}{N} \qquad (4-3)$$

And for the set of scores above:

$$AD = 6/5 = 1.2$$

Standard Deviation (*s*)

A second approach is to compute the difference between each score and the mean and then square these difference scores. This also produces a positive number that may be divided. If we divide this sum by $N - 1$ and take the square root of the quotient, we have a **standard deviation** (s):

$$s = \sqrt{\frac{\Sigma(X - \overline{X})^2}{N - 1}} \qquad (4\text{--}4)$$

Again, using the set of scores above:

X	$X - \overline{X}$	$|X - \overline{X}|$	$(X - \overline{X})^2$	X^2
1	-2	2	4	1
2	-1	1	1	4
3	0	0	0	9
4	1	1	1	16
5	2	2	4	25
	0	6	10	55

$$s = \sqrt{\frac{10}{4}} = \sqrt{2.5}$$

Formula 4.4 allows us to see what the standard deviation is and is easy to use as long as the scores and the mean are all whole numbers. But if the scores and/or the mean have several decimal places, computing and squaring the difference scores become troublesome. For this reason the following computational formula is usually preferred in calculating s:

$$s = \sqrt{\frac{\Sigma X^2 - \dfrac{(\Sigma X)^2}{N}}{N - 1}} \qquad (4\text{--}5)$$

For our data:

$$s = \sqrt{\frac{55 - \dfrac{(15)^2}{5}}{4}} = \sqrt{2.5}$$

Formulas 4.4 and 4.5 give us numerically the same answer, and formula 4.5 can be derived algebraically from 4.4.

Measures of Variability—Grouped Data

Semi-interquartile Range

Using the data in Table 3.1, we will consider how to compute Q and s when we have grouped data rather than individual raw scores. First the computation of Q.

In order to compute Q we must first determine Q_1 and Q_3. The procedure here is the same as that used in computing the median for these data. Q_1 is defined as that point in the distribution with $\frac{1}{4}$ of N of the scores falling below it, or for our data:

$$\tfrac{1}{4}(32,400) = 8,100$$

We see that there are 6,800 infants weighing less than 3,000.5 grams and that there are 12,000 infants weighing between 3,000.5 and 3,500.5 grams so that the 8100th score falls within this interval. Thus we need 1,300 of these 12,000 scores $(8,100 - 6,800 = 1,300)$.

$$Q_1 = 3,000.5 + \frac{1,300}{12,000}(500) = 3,054.7$$

In a similar fashion Q_3 is defined as that point in the distribution with $\frac{3}{4}$ of the N scores falling below it, or in this case:

$$\tfrac{3}{4}(32,400) = 24,300$$

18,800 infants weigh less than 3,500.5 grams; so we need $24,300 - 18,000 = 5,500$ more scores out of the next interval. Therefore:

$$Q_3 = 3,500.5 + \frac{5,500}{10,000}(500) = 3,775.5$$

Thus:

$$Q = \frac{3775.5 - 3054.7}{2} = 360.4$$

Standard Deviation

We are confronted with the same problem in computing the standard deviation for grouped data that we faced when we calculated the mean for these data, and the solution is the same: we use the midpoint (MP) of each interval as an estimate of all the scores in that interval. In formula 4.5 we computed the sum of all the raw scores (ΣX) and the sum of each score squared (ΣX^2). When we have grouped data we replace each raw score (X) with the midpoint of the interval in which the score falls, so that the sum of all the scores in an interval is $f(MP)$, and if we square each score in the interval and sum these, we have $f(MP^2)$. So the formula for grouped data is:

$$s = \sqrt{\frac{\Sigma f(MP^2) - \dfrac{(\Sigma fMP)^2}{N}}{N - 1}} \qquad (4\text{–}6)$$

Referring again to Table 3.2, summing column #4 produces $\Sigma f(MP)$ and summing column #5 gives us $\Sigma f(MP^2)$ so that:

$$s = \sqrt{\frac{380{,}884{,}458{,}100 - \dfrac{(109{,}466{,}200)^2}{32{,}400}}{32{,}399}} = 583.8$$

Measures of Variability and Scales of Measurement

When we were deciding what measure of central tendency to use we found that the first thing that we had to consider was the scale of measurement used in collecting the data. Since the scale of measurement determines what mathematical manipulations may be performed on the data we must also consider the scale of measurement used when we wish to compute a measure of variability.

If we have nominal scale data, the only way that we can indicate variability is to give the number of groups that have been used: patients were classified into four groups on the basis of blood type. If we have ordinal scale data, we assume a continuum and hence can order scores finding the largest and the smallest and thus can compute a range or, better still, Q. If we have equal units of measurement, an interval scale, then we can take square roots so we may compute an average deviation or a standard deviation.

Measures of Variability and Normal Distributions

In cases where our data are normally distributed, if we compute the median and add and subtract one Q from it, we will have a range that includes approximately 50% of the scores. For example, if $Md = 60$ and $Q = 10$, then 50% of the scores will fall within the interval 50 to 70 provided that the scores are normally distributed. Similarly if we compute the mean and add and subtract $1s$ from it, we will have an interval that includes approximately 68% of the scores; $\overline{X}$ plus and minus $2s$ includes approximately 95% of the scores; and $\overline{X}$ plus and minus $3s$ includes approximately 99% of the scores. These relationships hold only for normally distributed data.

Standard Scores

Now that we have an understanding of the mean and standard deviation, we can make use of these in computing standard scores. A **standard score** is the difference between a person's raw score and the mean expressed in standard deviation units:

$$\text{Standard score} = \frac{X - \overline{X}}{s} \qquad (4\text{-}7)$$

Standard scores have many uses, and any set of scores may be converted to standard scores. One reason for standardizing a set of scores is to convert them to a mean and standard deviation that are whole numbers. This is accomplished by multiplying the standard score by the new standard deviation we wish the scores to have and then adding the new mean to this value:

$$\text{Standard score} = \frac{X - \overline{X}}{s} \text{ (new } s) + \text{new } \overline{X} \qquad (4\text{-}8)$$

For example, if we wish to standardize a set of scores so that they have a mean of 100 and a standard deviation of 20, we would do this using the formula:

$$\text{Standard score} = \frac{X - \overline{X}}{s} (20) + 100$$

The means and standard deviations of many widely used tests have been standardized so that these values are whole numbers, for example, mean IQ $= 100$, mean GRE $= 500$.

The goal then in standardizing a set of scores is to change the mean and the standard deviation of the set of scores to some new values. It should be emphasized that standardizing scores does not change the shape of the distribution. If we start with a set of scores that has a skewed distribution, it will still be skewed after standardizing.

One standard score is encountered so frequently that it is given a special designation—a z score. A **z score** is a score that has been standardized with reference to a mean of zero and a standard deviation of one:

$$z = \frac{X - \overline{X}}{s} (1) + 0 = \frac{X - \overline{X}}{s} \qquad (4\text{-}9)$$

Furthermore, if the raw scores are normally distributed, then the z scores will be normally distributed and the distribution of z scores is called a **unit normal distribution.** Since this distribution has many applications, tables have been generated to give the various areas under this curve. Appendix A is such a table. Column #1 in this table lists the z scores; column #2 gives the area under the curve from the mean to z; column #3 lists the area under the curve in the larger portion; and column #4 gives the area under the smaller portion. (Since the distribution is symmetrical, only the right half of the curve is tabled.)

Suppose we have an IQ test with $\overline{X} = 100$ and $s = 20$ and a patient has a score of 127 on this test. Assuming that IQ is normally distributed, we can compute a z score and use Appendix A.

$$z = \frac{127 - 100}{20} = 1.35$$

Looking up $z = 1.35$ in column #1 tells us that 91% of the population have IQs of 127 or less (column #3) and that 9% have IQ's greater than 127 (column #4). Let us stress again that this is true only if the set of scores under consideration is normally distributed.

Exercise 4

Using the data for incubation periods in Exercise 3, calculate the range, semi-interquartile range, and standard deviation.

Chapter 5

Correlation: Pearson's *r*

So far we have limited our discussion to the task of describing one set of data. Correlation may be used to describe a relationship between two or more sets of data. Correlations are classified as either linear or curvilinear depending upon the nature of the relationship between the two sets of data.

If an investigator is considering the use of a correlation, the first thing that he or she should do is make a scatterplot of the data. A scatterplot is made by plotting one variable (*X*) on the abscissa of a graph, the second variable (*Y*) on the ordinate, and entering the data points on the figure. If the points on the scatterplot seem to approximate a straight line, then a linear correlation coefficient would be called for; if the points do not approximate a straight line, then we would use a curvilinear correlation coefficient (see Figure 5.1).

Linear Correlation Coefficients

We will begin by limiting our discussion to linear correlation coefficients. All linear correlation coefficients vary between $+1.0$ and -1.0, and all of them tell us two things. First, the sign of the correlation ($+$ or $-$) tells us how

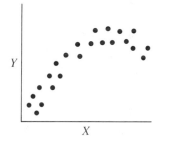

Figure 5.1. *Scatterplot of curvilinear data*

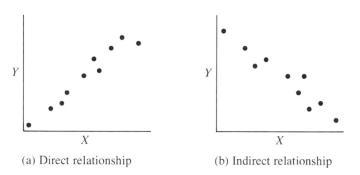

(a) Direct relationship   (b) Indirect relationship

Figure 5.2. *Scatterplots showing direct and indirect relationships*

the two sets of data are related. Figure 5.2a shows a scatterplot with the data approximating a straight line that rises from left to right. A correlation computed on these data would be positive since the relationship between X and Y is direct, in other words, as scores increase on X they tend to increase on Y also. Figure 5.2b, on the other hand, shows a linear trend that goes down from left to right. As scores get larger on X they also tend to get smaller on Y; so the data are inversely related, and a correlation computed on these data would be negative.

The second thing that any linear correlation coefficient tells us is the amount of variance that can be accounted for by a straight line. This information is provided by the numerical value of the correlation. A correlation of 0 tells us that there is no systematic relationship between X and Y. If we make a scatterplot of data that have a 0 correlation, it would look something like Figure 5.3. The data points appear at random on the graph, and if we enclose them with a line, we have a large circle.

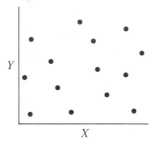

Figure 5.3.   *Scatterplot when correlation is zero*

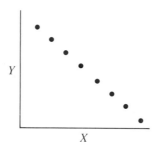

Figure 5.4.   *Scatterplot of correlation of negative one*

At the other extreme is a correlation of $+1.0$ or -1.0. A correlation with a value of 1 tells us that we have a perfect relationship, that is, we can draw a straight line through all the points on our scatterplot. Figure 5.4 is an example of data that would produce a correlation of -1.0.

On the two extremes then we have a correlation of 0, indicating no relationship between X and Y, and a correlation of 1.0, denoting a perfect linear correlation. Most data produce correlations in between these two extremes. If we looked at a series of relationships that ranged from 0 to $+1.0$, we would see that the scatterplots become narrower as we approach $+1.0$ (Figure 5.5).

At this point let us stress again that when one is considering the use of a correlation coefficient the first thing to do is to make a scatterplot. From this we can tell whether a linear or curvilinear correlation is appropriate. If the data are linearly related, we can tell whether the relationship is direct or inverse and we can estimate the magnitude of the correlation coefficient.

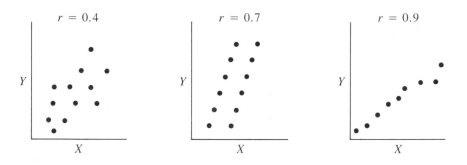

Figure 5.5. *Scatterplots of linear data*

Pearson's *r*

There are several different linear correlation coefficients, each designed for use in a specific situation. Pearson's product moment correlation coefficient, usually referred to as **Pearson's *r*** or more simply *r*, is the most frequently encountered linear correlation coefficient. It is used when we have two sets of data (*X* and *Y*) which are linearly related and both of which have been measured on at least an interval scale. There are many different formulas that may be used to compute *r* for a set of data. We will consider two of these. The first, formula 5.1, is usually referred to as a theoretical formula.

$$r = \frac{\Sigma(X - \overline{X})(Y - \overline{Y})}{\sqrt{\Sigma(X - \overline{X})^2 \Sigma(Y - \overline{Y})^2}} \qquad (5\text{–}1)$$

Like formula 4.3 for *s*, this formula gives us insight into the workings of *r* but is very difficult to use for most calculations. The numerator of 5.1 determines the sign of *r* (the denominator is a square root and we do not work with imaginary numbers in statistics), so let us look at it. It tells us that we have two sets of scores (*X* and *Y*), that we are to compute the means for both of these sets ($\overline{X}$ and $\overline{Y}$), that we are to take each pair of scores and subtract $\overline{X}$ from the *X* score and $\overline{Y}$ from the *Y* score, that we are to multiply these difference scores together for each pair, and finally that we are to sum these products. If we have a direct relationship between *X* and *Y*, then scores above the mean on *X* will tend to be paired with scores above the mean on *Y* so that $X - \overline{X}$ will be positive and $Y - \overline{Y}$ will be positive. When we multiply positive numbers together we obtain a positive product. Likewise, scores below the mean on *X* will tend to be paired with scores below the mean on Y so that $X - \overline{X}$ will be negative and $Y - \overline{Y}$ will be negative and when we multiply these two nega-tive numbers together we get a positive product too. When we sum all these positive numbers together we get a positive numerator.

If the relationship between X and Y is inverse, then scores above the mean on X tend to be paired with scores below the mean on Y, and vice versa; so $X - \overline{X}$ will be positive and $Y - \overline{Y}$ will be negative. When we multiply a posi-tive number times a negative number we obtain a negative product and hence a negative numerator.

As stated, formula 5.1 allows us to see why r may be positive or negative, but it is difficult to use in most situations. This is especially true if the scores and the means involve decimals that have to be squared and then multiplied together. Formula 5.2 is the raw score formula for calculating r and is pre-ferable to 5.1 for actual calculations:

$$r = \frac{N\Sigma XY - \Sigma X(\Sigma Y)}{\sqrt{\{N\Sigma X^2 - (\Sigma X)^2\}\{N\Sigma Y^2 - (\Sigma Y)^2\}}} \qquad (5\text{--}2)$$

We have encountered most of the notation used in formula 5.2 in our dis-cussion of s except that here we are working with two sets of scores. The sum of the cross products (ΣXY) is really the only new symbol in this formula. Suppose that we have the heights and weights of five patients and we wish to compute r for these data. To compute ΣXY we would multiply each patient's height by his weight and then sum these five products. N in this formula refers to the number of pairs of scores and not the actual number of raw scores. In our height–weight example $N = 5$ for the five patients even though there are ten scores (5 heights, 5 weights).

Consider the following example. An investigator has given ten rats IP in-jections of a drug (mg/kg) and then measured plasma levels of the drug (mg/ml) one hour later, generating the data in Table 5.1. When we plot the data (Figure 5.6) we see that: (1) it appears to be linear, (2) the correlation will be positive, and (3) it is of moderate magnitude.

By summing column #2 in Table 5.1 we find that $\Sigma X = 44$ and the sum of column #3 gives us $\Sigma Y = 4.6$. In column #4 we have squared each value of X, and column #5 has each Y^2. Summing these two columns produces $\Sigma X^2 = 238$ and $\Sigma Y^2 = 2.7$, respectively. Column #6 contains each of the cross products, and summing this column gives us $\Sigma XY = 23.9$. Substituting these values into formula 5.2 we have:

$$r = \frac{10(23.9) - 44(4.6)}{\sqrt{\{10(238) - (44)^2\}\{10(2.7) - (4.6)^2\}}} = .719$$

Table 5.1. *Dose–response data for drug experiment*

Subject #	Dosage (mg/kg) X	Plasma Level (mg/ml) Y	X^2	Y^2	XY
1	1.0	0.2	1	.04	.2
2	2.0	0.1	4	.01	.2
3	3.0	0.3	9	.09	.9
4	3.0	0.6	9	.36	1.8
5	4.0	0.2	16	.04	.8
6	5.0	0.5	25	.25	2.5
7	5.0	0.6	25	.36	3.0
8	6.0	0.9	36	.81	5.4
9	7.0	0.5	49	.25	3.5
10	8.0	0.7	64	.49	5.6
	44.0	4.6	238	2.7	23.9

mn 4.4

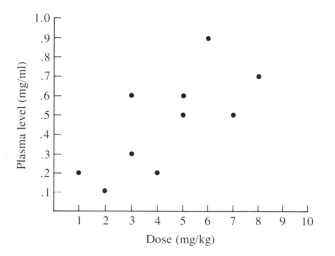

Figure 5.6. *Dose–response scatterplot of drug data*

Assumptions

It was noted earlier that the use of Pearson's *r* presupposes: (1) that X and Y are interval scale variables and (2) that they are linearly related. In addition X and Y should both be normally distributed continuous variables and their scatterplot should show homoscedasticity. **Homoscedasticity** means that we have arrays with equal variances. An array is simply a column of numbers; so if our scatterplot appears to be egg-shaped or cigar-shaped, we assume that this condition has been satisfied. If any of these four conditions are not met and we compute *r* for the data, we will end up with a correlation value that is numerically lower than if we had used some other correlation coefficient that is more appropriate for these data. Other types of correlations are discussed in Chapter 8. Computed correlations that are numerically lower than what actually exists in the data are referred to as being **spuriously low.** Spuriously low correlation coefficients may be produced if we violate any of the assumptions for the correlation or if we truncate the range of one or both variables. If we compute *r* for all the data in Figure 5.7, we would expect a large, positive *r*. However, suppose we limit our data to pairs of scores where $X \geq 5$. The scatterplot for this part of the data would indicate a correlation of close to zero.

Correlations between grade point average and IQ for medical or dental students are usually of low magnitude because by the time students are admitted to these programs the screening processes have eliminated everyone on the lower ends of these two scales.

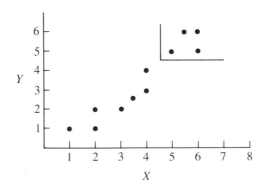

Figure 5.7.   *Effects of truncating the range of a correlation*

Causality

Correlation does not imply causality! That is, just because X and Y have a high correlation we can not assume that X causes Y, or vice versa. Two variables have a high correlation because they vary together in some systematic fashion. This may be because one "causes" the other, or it may be because both are under the influence of a third variable. If we are interested in determining what causes X, we may use correlation as a starting point in our investigation by taking measurements on a number of variables and correlating each of these with X. Variables that correlate highly with X would be investigated further in a systematic manner, while ones that have a low correlation with X would be discarded.

Exercise 5

For the data given below: (1) make a scatterplot and (2) compute Pearson's r.

X	Y
3	10
3	20
4	5
4	35
5	20
5	30
5	35
7	20
7	50
8	30
8	50
9	30
9	60
10	45
10	55
11	35
12	55
12	75
13	60
13	70

Chapter 6
Linear Regression

In the preceding chapter we saw that correlation may be used to show that some type of relationship exists between two variables. If this relationship is sufficiently large, we might want to capitalize on it and try to predict one variable from the other. For example, suppose that we find that a large positive correlation exists between high school science grades and freshman year nursing students' grades. We would like to use this relationship then to predict a student's performance in nursing school based upon his or her high school grades. This can be done if we can find the regression equation relating these two sets of scores.

Regression of Y on X

You may recall that the equation for a straight line is:

$$Y = a + bX \tag{6-1}$$

where a is the y intercept and b is the slope of the line. In this equation Y is the **dependent variable,** the one we wish to predict, and X is the **independent variable,** the one we know.

Let us use the dose-response data in Table 5.1. We computed Pearson's r for these data and found it to be 0.72. Now we would like to find the equation of the line that best fits these data so that for any dosage of the drug (X) we can predict the resulting plasma level (Y). In order to do this we must find the constants a and b in the above equation. We may solve for b by using the formula:

$$b_{yx} = \frac{N\Sigma XY - (\Sigma X)(\Sigma Y)}{N\Sigma X^2 - (\Sigma X)^2} \tag{6-2}$$

We have already computed ΣXY, ΣX, ΣY, ΣX^2, and ΣY^2 in finding r, and these are found in Table 5.1. Substituting these values into formula 6.2 we have:

$$b_{yx} = \frac{10(23.9) - 44(4.6)}{10(238) - 44} = .08$$

a may be found using the equation:

$$\overline{Y} = a + b\overline{X} \tag{6-3}$$

Thus:

$$.46 = a + .08(4.4)$$

$$a_{yx} = .11$$

Substituting the values that we have found into equation 6.1 for a and b we have:

$$\hat{Y} = .11 + .08X \tag{6-4}$$

The symbol $\hat{Y}$, called "Y hat," is used to indicate that the Y value is a predicted value and has not actually been measured.

Now that we have the regression equation, we may take any dose and by substituting it for X in equation 6.4, predict what the resulting plasma level $(\hat{Y})$ will be. If we have only a few values of X for which we wish to predict Y or if we have a computer available, we may substitute each X into the regression equation and solve for $\hat{Y}$. If, however, we have a large number of X's for which we want $\hat{Y}$'s and we do not have access to a computer, it is best to plot the regression line accurately on graph paper and make our predictions from the graph.

In order to plot the regression line, we pick two extreme values of X, substitute them into the regression equation, and solve for $\hat{Y}$. The resulting two points are then plotted and joined with a straight line. In the case of our dose-response data we could chose X values of 1 and 8. Substituting $X = 1$ into equation 6.4, we find $\hat{Y} = .19$; substituting $X = 8$, we find $\hat{Y} = .75$. Next we plot the points (1, .19) and (8, .75) and draw a line through these points. Now we can predict $\hat{Y}$ for any value of X simply by reading from X on the abscissa to the regression line and over to the Y axis.

Regression of X on Y

When we calculate Pearson's r it does not matter which variable we designate X or which is Y; the resulting value for r will be the same either way. This is not the case when we consider regression. We have already distinguished between independent and dependent variables in regression, and the foregoing example dealt with the case where X was independent and Y dependent. Suppose that now we wish to predict the initial dosage of the drug from the plasma level after one hour (X is now dependent, Y independent). If we interchange X's and Y's in formulas 6.1, 6.2, and 6.3, we will have the necessary equations. The slope constant is:

$$b_{xy} = \frac{N\Sigma XY - (\Sigma X)(\Sigma Y)}{N\Sigma Y^2 - (\Sigma Y)^2} \tag{6-5}$$

and for our example:

$$b_{xy} = \frac{10(23.9) - 44(4.6)}{10(2.7) - 4.6^2} = 6.17$$

The X intercept is:

$$\overline{X} = a + b\overline{Y} \tag{6-6}$$

or

$$4.4 = a + 6.17(.46)$$

$$a_{xy} = 1.56$$

The resulting regression equation for X as the dependent variable is:

$$\hat{X} = 1.56 + 6.17Y \tag{6-7}$$

Let us now pick two extreme values for Y and solve for the corresponding values of $\hat{X}$. If $Y = .1$, we find that $\hat{X} = 2.18$, and for $Y = .8$, $\hat{X} = 6.5$. These two points have also been plotted in Figure 6.1.

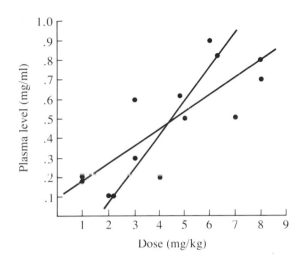

Figure 6.1.   *Scatterplot and regression lines*

Standard Error of Estimate

If we have a perfect correlation ($r = \pm 1$), all of the data points will be on the regression line and we will be able to predict exactly any value of the dependent variable. In fact, correlations are rarely perfect, so that there will be error involved in our predictions. Suppose we have a group of 40 students and we randomly pick 20 of these students, measure their heights and weights, compute r, and solve the regression equation with height as the independent variable. Now we can go back to the remaining 20 students, ask each his height (X), and then predict his weight ($\hat{Y}$) on the basis of the regression equation. In this case we could also measure each of the 20 students so that we would have both Y and $\hat{Y}$. The difference between Y and $\hat{Y}$ for each student then is error and describes how scores may vary about the regression line. These difference scores are incorporated into a statistic called a **standard error of estimate** (s_{yx}) defined as:

$$s_{yx} = \sqrt{\frac{\Sigma(Y - \hat{Y})^2}{N - 2}} \qquad (6\text{--}8)$$

You will note that this formula looks very similar to the formula for s, and in fact its use is very similar: s measures how scores vary about the mean, and s_{yx} measures how scores vary about a regression line.

In the real world when regression is used we usually do not know what the actual values for the dependent variable are. If we have determined the regression equation between high school science GPA and freshman nursing GPA's and want to predict Sue Jones' GPA at the end of her freshman year of nursing school ($\hat{Y}$), we can do that now but we will have to wait a year for her to complete her freshman year before we have Y. In situations like this the standard error of estimate may be calculated using the formula:

$$s_{yx} = s_y \sqrt{1 - r^2} \tag{6-9}$$

This is an estimate, and if r is based upon less than 50 pairs of observations, it should be multiplied by

$$\sqrt{\frac{N-1}{N-2}} \tag{6-10}$$

To return once again to our dose-response data in Table 5.1, the standard error of estimate for dose as the independent variable is

$$s_{yx} = .24\sqrt{1 - .72^2} \ \sqrt{\tfrac{9}{8}} = .19$$

Since there are two regression lines and since we have applied subscripts to the standard error of estimate, you have no doubt guessed that there are two standard errors of estimate, one for each regression line. To compute the standard error of estimate when Y is the independent variable, we interchange X's and Y's in formulas 6.8 and 6.9. Thus:

$$s_{xy} = \sqrt{\frac{\Sigma(X - \hat{X})^2}{N-2}} \tag{6-11}$$

$$s_{xy} = s_x \sqrt{1 - r^2} \tag{6-12}$$

For our dose-response data with plasma level as the independent variable we have:

$$s_{xy} = 2.11\sqrt{1 - .72^2} \ \sqrt{\tfrac{9}{8}} = 1.63$$

Exercise 6

Using the data in Exercise 5, compute the regression equation of X on Y and Y on X. Make a scatterplot of the data and plot the two regression lines on it. Compute s_{yx} and s_{xy}.

Chapter 7
Other Correlation Coefficients

In Chapter 6 we considered Pearson's product moment correlation coefficient, noting that it is the most commonly encountered linear correlation coefficient. In this chapter we will look at a number of other linear correlation coefficients and end the chapter with a discussion of a curvilinear correlation.

Other Linear Correlations

Rho ρ

In order to determine if any relationship exists between severity of emphysema symptoms and smoking, Dr. E. asks each of eight patients attending the lung clinic on a particular day how much he or she smokes. Another physician ranks the eight patients with regard to the severity of their illness. Here we have one set of data that is ordinal scale (severity of illness) and one set that is ratio scale (number of cigarettes smoked per day). One correlation that will handle this combination is Spearman's rank order correlation coefficient, or rho, which is designed for two sets of ranks. Thus we can rank the patients with regard to the amount that they smoke and compute rho using this formula:

$$\rho = 1 - \frac{6\Sigma D^2}{N(N^2 - 1)} \qquad (7\text{--}1)$$

where D is the difference in a pair of ranks. Using the data in Table 7.1 we have:

$$\rho = 1 - \frac{6(24)}{8(63)} = .715$$

In using rho one must be careful that ranks are assigned the same way to both variables, that is, if a rank of #1 indicates the person who smokes the least, then a rank of #1 should indicate the person with the least severe symptoms. If this is not done consistently for both variables, the sign of the correlation coefficient will be reversed.

Table 7.1. *Amount smoked and severity of illness*

Patient #	Amount Smoked (rank)	Severity of Illness (rank)	D	D^2
1	6	5	−1	1
2	7	8	1	1
3	2	4	2	4
4	3	3	0	0
5	5	7	2	4
6	4	1	−3	9
7	1	2	1	1
8	8	6	−2	4
				$24 = \Sigma D^2$

Point biserial (r_{pb})

The point biserial correlation is used when one variable is continuous and the other variable is a true dichotomy. Suppose that Dr. H is testing the possible carcinogenic effect of a lipstick coloring. He applies this compound to varying amounts of the body surface of some rats and after a month examines the animals. Since the amount of body surface exposed can vary from 0% to

100%, it is a continuous variable, and on the day of the exam the rat either has skin cancer or does not; so this variable is a true dichotomy. To determine if any relationship exists between amount of exposure and the presence or absence of cancer, Dr. H may use the point biserial correlation.

$$r_{pb} = \frac{\overline{X}_p - \overline{X}_t}{s_t} \sqrt{\frac{N_p N_t}{N_0(N_t - 1)}} \qquad (7\text{--}2)$$

where:

$\overline{X}_p$ = mean area of exposure for animals developing cancer

$\overline{X}_t$ = mean area of exposure of all animals

s_t = standard deviation of area of exposure of all animals

N_p = number of animals developing cancer

N_0 = number of animals who did not develop cancer

$N_t = N_p + N_0$

Let us suppose that Dr. H decided to divide 70 animals into 4 groups: 10 animals received no exposure, 25 had a 25% exposure, 25 had a 50% exposure, and 10 had a 90% exposure. The results are recorded in Table 7.2. In order to compute r_{pb} we must first determine:

$$N_p = 39 \qquad\qquad N_0 = 31 \qquad\qquad N_t = 70$$

$$\overline{X}_t = 2775/70 = 39.64 \qquad \overline{X}_p = 2060/39 = 52.82$$

$$s_t = \sqrt{\frac{159{,}125 - (2775)^2/70}{69}} = 26.49$$

then

$$r_{pb} = \frac{52.82 - 39.64}{26.49} \sqrt{\frac{39(70)}{31(69)}} = .562$$

Table 7.2.   *Incidence of cancer in exposed rats*

% Body Area Exposed	Number Developing Cancer	Total Number			
X	f_p	f_t	$f_t(X)$	$f_t(X)^2$	$f_p(X)$
0	0	10	0	0	0
25	10	25	625	15,625	250
50	20	25	1250	62,500	1000
90	9	10	900	81,000	810
	39	70	2775	159,125	2060

Biserial r_b

In situations where both variables are continuous variables but one has been forced into a dichotomy, we use a biserial correlation coefficient. If we wanted to correlate the scores that students received on their anatomy final with whether they passed or failed the course, we could use this coefficient. Whether a student passes the course depends upon the total number of points that he or she accumulates during the quarter. If he or she is above the cut-off point, he or she passes so that the continuous variable "total number of points" has been forced into a pass-fail dichotomy.

The formula for the biserial correlation is:

$$r_b = \frac{\overline{X}_p - \overline{X}_t}{s_t}(p/y) \qquad (7\text{--}3)$$

where the terms are defined as in formula 7.2. p is the proportion of individuals that are positive, and y is the height of the ordinate cutting off an area equal to p above it on the normal curve.

If we use the numbers in Table 7.2 to compute r_b, we would obtain y by entering Appendix A and going down column #3 till we find $p = 39/70 = .56$. Then reading across to column #5 we find that $y = .3945$; so

$$r_b = \frac{52.82 - 39.64}{26.49}\left(\frac{.56}{.3945}\right) = .706$$

Phi ϕ

The phi coefficient is used when both of the variables under study are true dichotomies. The infirmary at the university took a random sample of 500 students and found that 218 of them had flu. Of the 500 students, 280 were males and the data are summarized in Table 7.3. A phi coefficient may be used to determine if any relationship exists between the incidence of flu and the sex of the patient.

If the cells in a 2 × 2 table are labeled A, B, C, and D and the row and column totals are designated J, K, L, and M, then the formula for phi is:

A	B	J
C	D	K
L	M	

$$\phi = \frac{AD - BC}{\sqrt{(J)(K)(L)(M)}} \qquad (7\text{--}4)$$

Table 7.3. *Incidence of flu by sex of patient*

	Flu	No Flu	
Males	118	162	280
Females	100	120	220
	218	282	500

so for our example we have

$$\phi = \frac{118(120) - 162(100)}{\sqrt{(280)(220)(218)(282)}} = -.033$$

The maximum size of phi is determined by how the two variables are split. In our example the row totals and column total are close to being evenly split, and in this case phi has a maximum of ± 1. As these totals deviate from a 50–50 split, the theoretical maximum that phi may assume is reduced.

Tetrachoric (r_{tet})

The tetrachoric correlation coefficient is designated for use when both of the variables are continuous but have been forced into dichotomies. This coefficient is obtained by solving a second-order quadratic equation, but since this may involve considerable work, computing devices have been developed. These result in approximate values for r_{tet}, and it is preferable to use phi in these situations.

Multiple $r_{1 \cdot 23}$

The multiple correlation coefficient makes use of information on three or more variables. If we are interested in predicting variable #1, then we look for a second variable (#2) that is correlated with #1. But suppose that we find a third variable (#3) that is also correlated with #1. Then perhaps if we combine #2 and #3, we will be able to predict #1 more accurately than by using either #2 or #3 separately. Whole books have been written on multiply correlation and regression describing how to maximize predictability by choice of variables, weighting of variables, etc. Here we will consider only the case of three variables, each variable being given equal weight.

If we want to know the correlation between variable #1 and the combination of variables #2 and #3, we may use the formula

$$r_{1\cdot23} = \sqrt{\frac{r_{12}^2 + r_{13}^2 - (2r_{12}r_{13}r_{23})}{1 - r_{23}^2}} \qquad (7\text{--}5)$$

If

$$\#1 = \text{Freshman GPA in college}$$
$$\#2 = \text{High school GPA}$$
$$\#3 = \text{College board exam score}$$

then we might like to know if combining high school GPA and college board exams will give us a higher correlation with college GPA than either high school GPA or college board exams will separately. We would collect information on these three variables for a group of students and suppose the resulting Pearson's r's to be:

$$r_{12} = .6$$
$$r_{13} = .7 \qquad \text{then} \qquad r_{1\cdot23} = \sqrt{\frac{.6^2 + .7^2 - (2)(.6)(.7)(.3)}{1 - .3^2}} = .81$$
$$r_{23} = .3$$

Note that in this example the resulting multiple correlation is larger than either r_{12} or r_{13}, so that the combination of #2 and #3 does give us more information than either variable taken separately. In selecting variables to be used in multiple correlation, one should look for independent variables that have high correlations with the dependent variable but low correlations with each other.

Partial $r_{12\cdot3}$

The partial correlation also makes use of information about three variables, but here the attempt is to partial out the effect of the third variable.

An investigator wants to look at the relationship between blood pressure and height for a group of patients, but after collecting his data he is concerned that any relationship between these two variables may be a function that both of these variables are related to weight. His computed Pearson's r's for each of the combinations are:

$$\#1 = \text{Blood pressure} \qquad r_{12} = .6$$
$$\#2 = \text{Height} \qquad r_{13} = .9$$
$$\#3 = \text{Weight} \qquad r_{23} = .7$$

The partial correlation will give our investigator the correlation between blood pressure and height with the effect of weight partialed out. The formula for the partial correlation coefficient is:

$$r_{12\cdot3} = \frac{r_{12} - r_{13}r_{23}}{\sqrt{(1 - r_{13}^2)(1 - r_{23}^2)}} \tag{7-6}$$

so

$$r_{12\cdot3} = \frac{.6 - (.9)(.7)}{\sqrt{(1 - .9^2)(1 - .7^2)}} = -.10$$

Here we see that a large positive correlation ($r_{12} = .6$) becomes a small negative correlation ($r_{12\cdot3} = -.10$) when the effect of a third variable is eliminated.

All of the correlation coefficients that have been discussed so far are linear correlation coefficients and vary between ± 1. We will now consider the correlation ratio, or eta, that is used with data that have a curvilinear relationship.

Curvilinear Correlation

Eta η

Dr. B designed the following study to investigate the relationship between stress and corticosterone. Fifty-seven rats were individually placed into a box where they received ten electric shocks. Each animal was randomly assigned to one of six groups and plasma corticosterone levels were measured for group I five minutes after the last shock, for group II sixty minutes after the last shock, for group III 120 minutes after the last shock, for group IV 240 minutes, for group V 480 minutes, and for group VI 960 minutes. The results are recorded in Table 7.4 and graphed in Figure 7.1. Inspection of this figure indicates that plasma corticosterone is elevated immediately after shock, that it decreases then, and that this is followed by an increase—a curvilinear relationship.

Designating plasma corticosterone as Y and time after shock as X, eta is defined as:

$$\eta_{yx} = \sqrt{\frac{\sum \left(\dfrac{Y_j^2}{n_j}\right) - \dfrac{(\sum Y_{ij})^2}{N}}{\sum Y_{ij}^2 = \dfrac{(\sum Y_{ij})^2}{N}}} \tag{7-7}$$

Table 7.4.   *Plasma corticosterone levels after shock*

Time after Last Shock in Minutes	5	60	120	240	480	960
	65	25	20	15	25	33
	63	24	20	13	24	30
	61	23	19	12	23	30
	61	22	19	12	22	29
	60	21	18	11	22	29
	60	21	17	11	20	28
	59	20	17	10	20	28
	59	20	16	10	19	27
	55	19	15	9	17	27
	50	18	15			
	593	213	176	103	192	261

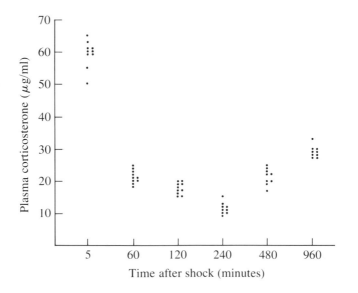

Figure 7.1.   *Plasma corticosterone levels after shock*

where:

n_j = the number of scores in column j

Y_j = the sum of the scores in column j

N = the total number of scores in the table

ΣY_{ij} = the sum of all the scores in the table with regard to Y

so that

$$\Sigma Y_{ij} = 65 + 63 + 61 + \cdot\,\cdot\,\cdot + 27 + 27 = 1538$$

$$\Sigma Y_{ij}^2 = 65^2 + 63^2 + 61^2 + \cdot\,\cdot\,\cdot + 27^2 + 27^2 = 55,984$$

$$N = 57$$

$$\frac{(\Sigma Y_{ij})^2}{N} = \frac{1538^2}{57} = 41,499$$

$$\Sigma\left(\frac{Y_j^2}{n_j}\right) = \frac{593^2 + 213^2 + 176^2}{10} + \frac{103^2 + 192^2 + 261^2}{9} = 55,643$$

$$\eta_{yx} = \sqrt{\frac{55,643 - 41,499}{55,984 - 41,499}} = .98$$

We have put subscripts on eta because for any given set of data two etas may be calculated. η_{xy} is obtained by substituting X's for Y's in formula 7.7. $\eta_{yx} \neq \eta_{xy}$.

In our discussion of linear correlation coefficients we indicated that these may vary between plus and minus one. Curvilinear correlations vary from zero to plus one; they do not take on negative values. The sign of the linear correlation coefficient tells us how X and Y are related, but if X and Y have a curvilinear relationship, then they may be directly related over part of their range and indirectly related over part of their range so that the sign has no meaning.

The standard error of estimate for eta may be computed as follows:

$$s_{\eta_{yx}} = \sqrt{\frac{\Sigma Y_{ij}^2 - \Sigma\left(\dfrac{Y_j^2}{n_j}\right)}{N - K}} \tag{7-8}$$

where:

k = the number of columns

Substituting X's for Y's in formula 7.8 will result in the standard error of estimate for η_{xy}.

Exercise 7

1. A researcher injected 16 mice with varying doses of a compound and measured the amount of the compound excreted in the following 24 hours. Compute eta for these data.

Amount Injected (mg/kg)	Amount Excreted
.1	.09
.1	.08
.2	.16
.2	.17
.5	.45
.5	.49
.75	.70
.75	.72
1.0	.85
1.0	.80
1.5	.85
1.5	.82
1.75	.87
1.75	.80
2.0	.83
2.0	.85

2. An investigator wished to know if congenital malformations were correlated with the age of the mother, so he selected 3000 birth certificates and obtained the following information. Use phi to see if there is a correlation.

	Malformation	No Malformation
Age: $\geq$ 35	21	1479
Age: $<$ 35	9	1491

3. Birth weight (gm) and age of mother (years) were recorded for 20 infants. Compute rho for these data.

Age		Birth Weight		d	d^2
15	[1]	2000	[2]	1	1
21	[7]	2400	[9.5]	2.5	6.25
26	[14.5]	4600	[18]	3.5	12.25
18	[3]	2100	[3.5]	0.5	0.25
31	[19]	5100	[20]	1	1
19	[4]	2200	[5.5]	1.5	2.25
22	[8.5]	2700	[11]	2.5	6.25
24	[11.5]	3200	[14]	2.5	6.25
20	[5.5]	2300	[7.5]	2	4
29	[18]	3000	[12]	6	36
25	[13]	4000	[16]	3	9
27	[16]	4500	[17]	1	1
23	[10]	2400	[9.5]	0.5	0.25
32	[20]	2200	[5.5]	14.5	210.25
24	[11.5]	3500	[15]	3.5	12.25
26	[14.5]	3100	[13]	1.5	2.25
20	[5.5]	1900	[1]	4.5	20.25
17	[2]	2100	[3.5]	1.5	2.25
28	[17]	5000	[19]	2	4
22	[8.5]	2300	[7.5]	1	1
					338

$$\rho = 1 - \frac{6\Sigma d^2}{N(N^2-1)} = 1 - \frac{6 \times 338}{20(400-1)} = 1 - \frac{2028}{7980} =$$

$$= 1 - .25 = .75$$

$$\rho + .75 < .01$$

Chapter 8
Sampling

In most situations it is impossible to measure every element in the population; so we are reduced to selecting a sample from the population, making measurements on that sample, and then making inferences about the population on the basis of our sample data. We define a **population** as the set of elements that we are interested in studying. Numerically the population may be very large or very small, such as all the registered nurses in the United States or all the neurosurgeons in Lincoln County. A **sample** is a subset of the population under study.

Nonprobability Samples

Samples may be chosen in a variety of ways and are classified as probability samples or nonprobability samples. **Nonprobability samples** are samples in which we can not specify what the chances are that a particular element in the population will be included in the sample. Suppose that you want to predict the outcome of the school election in Beaverbury and you go to the main intersection in that town and ask the first 20 registered voters you encounter how they will vote. It is impossible for you to determine what the chances are of selecting those particular 20 voters. This would be called an **accidental sample** because you have selected these 20 people by accident.

Another type of nonprobability sample is a **purposive sample.** Suppose I believe that I have developed a cure for the common cold and I wish to test it. I select 40 people who meet my criteria of "having a cold" and give 20 of them aspirin and 20 of them my wonder drug. Here I have purposively selected my sample and can not determine what the chances are that a given person will meet my criteria of a cold and be selected for the study.

Probability Samples

A probability sample is one in which we can determine what the odds are that a particular element in the population will be included in the sample. The most commonly encountered probability sample is a random sample. A **random sample** is one in which every element in the population has an equal and independent chance of being selected for the sample and each possible sample has an equal chance of being drawn. If we have a class of 100 students and we wish to draw a random sample of size ten, we could write each student's name on a 3×5 card, shuffle and cut this deck of cards, and take the top ten cards as our sample. Every student has an equal chance of being selected, and we can specify that the chance that any particular student will be included in the sample is $1/10$.

Stratified random samples and cluster samples are elaborations of simple random samples. Suppose that we wish to forecast the outcome of the election for governor of the state and because we feel that whether an individual is registered as a Democrat, a Republican, or an Independent is important to the outcome of the election, we wish these categories to appear in our sample with the same frequency as they appear in the population. If we select a large random sample, this would probably happen, but we are very limited by time and money so we are only going to sample 100 voters. We determine that of all the registered voters in the state 60% are Democrats, 30% Republicans, and 10% Independents. We obtain a list of all the registered Democrats and randomly select 60 for our study. Likewise we would randomly select 30 voters from the list of registered Republicans and 10 from the list of Independents. This is a **stratified random sample,** stratified with proportional allocation. We have identified a variable that we think is important for our study, stratified the population and the sample on the basis of this variable, and then randomly sampled from each strata.

It has recently been stated that parents are not having their children immunized for polio and that we may soon have an epidemic. You live in a town of 30,000 and want to see if this is true. You decide that the population for your study will be the grade-school children, and you obtain the names and addresses of all 7500 of these from the local school district office. If you randomly select 1000 of these names, you will have to run all over the town to track them down. An alternative that will save you time is to randomly select some number of city blocks, go to each block, and determine how many children on that block have been immunized by going from door-to-door. This is a **cluster sample.** The cluster, in this case all the children living on one city block, is randomly selected.

We can make the sampling scheme more elaborate by combining clustering and stratification. For example, in the foregoing study if we felt that socioeconomic level might influence whether a family sought immunization, we could stratify the town on the basis of socioeconomic levels and then randomly select blocks from each of these strata.

Parameters and Statistics

We have already indicated that the goal behind selecting a sample is to make a statement about the population. For example, we might compute the mean and standard deviation of our sample and wish to use these as estimates of the corresponding values in the population. To distinguish between values determined on the population and those determined on the sample, we refer to computations based upon the population as **parameters** and designate these with Greek letters, and those based upon the sample are called **statistics** and are designated with English letters. The mean of the population is given the symbol mu (μ), and its formula is:

$$\mu = \frac{\Sigma X}{N} \tag{8-1}$$

The sample mean is designated $\overline{X} = \Sigma X/N$.

The same procedure is used to compute μ and $\overline{X}$, the difference being that in the formula for μ, N is the whole population while in the formula for $\overline{X}$, N is something less than the whole population. In a similar fashion the sample standard deviation is designated by s and the corresponding parameter is σ.

$$\sigma = \sqrt{\frac{\Sigma X^2 - (\Sigma X)^2/N}{N}} \qquad (8\text{--}2)$$

$$s = \sqrt{\frac{\Sigma X^2 - (\Sigma X)^2/N}{N - 1}} \qquad (8\text{--}3)$$

Biased Samples

If our sample deviates in any systematic way from the population that we are trying to generalize to, we say that it is biased. Suppose you have heard that there is an outbreak of gastrointestinal illness among migrant workers in your county and wishing to substantiate this report, you randomly select 150 names out of the phone book, call these individuals, and ask if they have recently had any GI problems. The population under study is migrants, and we have a random sample of people with listed phone numbers. Since many migrants do not have phones, we have a random sample but not of the population that we are interested in studying.

Questionnaire sampling appears to be easy until we try it for the first time. It is obvious to the person writing the questions what information he is trying to obtain, but it is not always apparent to the respondent. Questionnaires should always be tested on a pilot group to clear up ambiguities. Questions should be stated as clearly and as briefly as possible. Attitudes cannot be equated to behavior. For example, asking "Do you believe smoking is harmful?" is not the same as asking "Do you smoke?" Nonrespondents are another problem. Usually they are ignored or assumed to be evenly divided into pros and cons. Research shows that with emotionally charged material neither of these approaches may be appropriate.

Sampling Distributions

Let us define the population under study as the 32,400 infants born in Oregon during 1972 and birth weight as the variable that we are studying. In this case we could eventually obtain all 32,400 raw scores and compute μ and σ. However, this is a costly procedure. So why not settle for a random sample of 100? We randomly select 100 birth certificates and compute the mean weight of these subjects, $\overline{X}_1$. Now suppose we repeat this process twice more and calculate $\overline{X}_2$ and $\overline{X}_3$. We would probably find that $\overline{X}_1 \neq \overline{X}_2 \neq \overline{X}_3$. Suppose that we continue drawing random samples and computing the means of these samples until we have 300 sample means. If we make a frequency polygon of these 300 sample means this would be a sampling distribution of the mean. The mean of this sampling distribution, in this case the mean of the sample means, should be equal to μ.

In the general case, if we draw a large number of random samples from a population, compute a statistic on each sample, and make a frequency polygon of the statistics, we will produce a **sampling distribution** for that statistic. In other words, all statistics have sampling distributions. If the mean of the sampling distribution of a statistic is equal to the corresponding parameter, we say that the statistic is an unbiased estimator of the parameter. We have pointed out that if we draw random samples, $\overline{X}$ is an unbiased estimator of μ because the mean of the sampling distribution of $\overline{X}$ is equal to μ.

If we compute s^2 for each of our 300 samples, we would find that the mean of these 300 sample variances would be equal to σ^2, that is, s^2 is an unbiased estimator of σ^2. If we wish to estimate σ from a sample, the statistic that we use is:

$$s = \sqrt{\frac{\Sigma X^2 - (\Sigma X)^2/N}{N - 1}} \qquad (8–4)$$

Standard Errors

We know that when we have a set of raw scores the mean describes the midpoint of the distribution and that the standard deviation describes how scores vary about that midpoint. With a sampling distribution we are working with statistics rather than raw scores, but as noted previously we can also compute a mean for the sampling distribution. If we wish to describe variability in the sampling distribution, then we are trying to describe how statistics vary about the mean of their sampling distribution. The variability of raw scores about their mean is given by the standard deviation; the variability of the statistic about the mean of its sampling distribution is given by the **standard error** of the statistic. All statistics have standard errors. The standard error of the mean ($s_{\overline{x}}$) is computed using the formula:

$$s_{\overline{x}} = s/\sqrt{N} = \sqrt{\frac{\Sigma X^2 - (\Sigma X)^2/N}{N(N - 1)}} \qquad (8–5)$$

This describes how sample means vary about μ.

Confidence Intervals

Suppose that we have randomly selected a sample of 50 healthy male medical students and measured their testosterone levels. The mean and standard error for our sample are $\overline{X} = 450$ ng/100ml and $s_{\overline{x}} = 70$ ng/100ml and we would like to estimate the mean for the total population, μ. Since we have a random sample we know that $\overline{X}$ is an unbiased estimate of μ, but we also know that it is very unlikely that $\overline{X} = \mu$ exactly. We can calculate a band of scores or a confidence interval that we feel reasonably sure will encompass μ. This is done using the formula:

$$z = \frac{\overline{X} - \mu}{s_{\overline{x}}} \qquad (8-6)$$

and rearranging it so that we have:

$$\overline{X} - zs_{\overline{x}} \leq \mu \leq \overline{X} + zs_{\overline{x}} \qquad (8-7)$$

$\overline{X}$ and $s_{\overline{x}}$ come from our sample, and z is obtained from the normal curve table in Appendix A. If we wish to compute a 99% confidence interval $z = 2.58$, and for a 95% confidence interval $z = 1.96$. Thus, for a 95% confidence interval for our example:

$$450 - (1.96)(70) \leq \mu \leq 450 + (1.96)(70)$$
$$312.8 \leq \mu \leq 587.2$$

We are 95% confident that the true population mean falls within the interval 312.8 to 587.2 ng/100ml.

Chapter 9
Probability

Most of us think of mathematics in terms of rules that prove a particular statement to be true or false, such as: "The sum of the angles of a triangle is 180°." Statistics, however, never proves anything in an absolute sense, and this is why when you read a journal article you come across statements like, "Therefore we conclude that diet A is better than diet B ($P \leq .05$)." The ($P \leq .05$) is really a qualifying statement saying that the author believes that diet A is better but that there is a probability of 5 in 100 that the findings may have been the result of chance errors. All inferential statistical tests are based upon probability, and all conclusions are made at a given probability level. This probability level is set by the investigator and is determined by how rigorous he or she wishes to be in a particular situation.

While all inferential statistics are based upon probability, it is possible for a person to use statistics for years and never have to actually compute a probability because of the various statistical tables that are available. However, if researchers are confronted with small samples they may find the direct application of probability not only useful but mandatory. In addition, a small brush with probability theory helps us to better appreciate the probability statements associated with all inferential statistics.

Probability

First let us define **probability** as the expected frequency with which an event occurs or as the proportion of all possible events that are of a particular type. The probability that we will flip a true coin and get a head is $\frac{1}{2}$ since there are two possible outcomes and only one of these is a head.

Probability Rules

Second, we must note that there are two rules for computing probabilities. The **multiplication rule** states that: the probability of the occurrence of two or more independent events is given by the product of their separate probabilities. The **addition rule** states that: the probability of the occurrence of two or more mutually exclusive events is the sum of their separate probabilities. (Two events are considered to be independent if the outcome of the first in no way influences the outcome of the second. Two events are mutually exclusive if when one occurs the other can not occur.) In either case, we must first determine the probability of each of the events. Then if the events are independent, we multiply these probabilities; if they are mutually exclusive we add them.

What is the probability of flipping a true coin twice and getting heads both times? The probability of a head on the first flip is $\frac{1}{2}$; the probability of a head on the second flip is $\frac{1}{2}$. What happens on the first flip does not influence what happens on the second flip, so the two events are independent. Hence the probability of two heads in two flips is: $(\frac{1}{2})(\frac{1}{2}) = \frac{1}{4}$.

What is the probability of cutting an ace or a king from a deck of well-shuffled cards? There are 4 aces and 4 kings in a deck of 52 cards; so the probability of cutting an ace is $4/52$ and the probability of cutting a king is $4/52$. If we cut a king we can not cut an ace, and vice versa; so the two events are mutually exclusive, and hence the probability of cutting either an ace or a king is $4/52 + 4/52 = 2/13$.

Binomial Experiments

Now that we have the basic principles, let us see how these are applied in binomial experiments. **Binomial experiments** are experiments composed of n independent trials, each trial having only two possible outcomes. Suppose that you are an obstetrician and that you have 10 patients who have been taking a particular brand of birth-control pill for two or more years and who just have had their first child. The results of these 10 pregnancies are 8 girls and 2 boys, and the thought occurs to you that perhaps this brand of pill might influence the sex of the children born to women who take it. To evaluate this proposition, you must first determine the probability of 8 girls in 10 births, assuming that only chance is operating. Second, you must decide if this event would occur frequently enough by chance alone that the pill is not responsible or if it would occur so infrequently by chance that the pill did play a role.

Each woman can have a boy or a girl, and the sex of each woman's child is independent of the sex of the others; so we have a binomial experiment consisting of 10 trials. Our first task is to determine the probability of 8 or more girls being born in 10 births. There are several possible ways that we can do this. One way would be to list all the possible sequences of 10 births starting with 10 girls, 0 boys, and going through 0 girls, 10 boys; then count the number of sequences that would result in 8 or more girls; and put this over the total number of sequences. Since there are 1024 different sequences that could result from 10 births, this method is not too practical in this situation.

Permutations

A second possible way to approach binomial experiments is through the use of permutations. **Permutations** are ordered sequences. The number of possible permutations of n objects taken n at a time is given by:

$$_nP_n = n! \qquad (9-1)$$

If I have five students and I want to know how many different lists I could construct using their names:

$$_nP_n = {}_5P_5 = 5! = (5)(4)(3)(2)(1) = 120$$

Sometimes we do not wish to use all the objects but want to construct permutations of r objects from a group of n objects; so we use the formula:

$$_nP_r = \frac{n!}{(n-r)!} \qquad (9-2)$$

If I had a class of 10 students and wanted to know how many permutations of size five I could draw from this class:

$$_{10}P_5 = \frac{10!}{(10-5)!} = 30{,}240$$

To return to our problem, some of the objects are indistinguishable, that is, we have girl babies and boy babies. Where we have indistinguishable objects which we designate $r_1, r_2, \ldots, r_k$, the number of permutations is given by:

$$_nP_{r_1, r_2, \ldots, r_k} = \frac{n!}{r_1! \, r_2! \cdots r_k!} \tag{9-3}$$

Now we can solve our problem. There is one sequence of 10 births that will give us 10 girls, 0 boys:

$$_{10}P_{10,0} = \frac{10!}{10!} = 1$$

There are 10 sequences that will result in 9 girls and 1 boy:

$$_{10}P_{9,1} = \frac{10!}{9! \, 1!} = 10$$

and there are 45 sequences that will result in 8 girls, 2 boys:

$$_{10}P_{8,2} = \frac{10!}{8! \, 2!} = 45$$

If we have 8 girls and 2 boys, we can not have 9 girls and 1 boy or 10 girls, so these outcomes are mutually exclusive. Since there are 1024 possible sequences, the probability of observing 8 or more girls in 10 births is:

$$1/1024 + 10/1024 + 45/1024 = 56/1024 = .0547$$

Binomial Theorem

A third way to solve a binomial experiment is to use the binomial theorem. If we let p be the probability that the event will happen, q the probability that the event will not happen and n the number of trials, we can expand the binomial:

$$(p+q)^n = p^n + np^{n-1}q + \frac{n(n-1)}{2!} p^{n-2}q^2 \tag{9-4}$$

$$+ \frac{n(n-1)(n-2)}{3!} p^{n-3}q^3 + \cdots + q^n$$

In our example p is the probability of having a girl, q is the probability of having a boy, and $n = 10$. Since we want to know the probability of having eight or more girls we are only interested in the first three terms of the binomial expansion which are:

$$\tfrac{1}{2}^{10} + 10(\tfrac{1}{2})^9(\tfrac{1}{2}) + 45(\tfrac{1}{2})^8(\tfrac{1}{2})^2 = 1/1024 + 10/1024 + 45/1024 = .0547$$

z Scores

A fourth solution of binomial experiments may be approximated using z scores and the normal curve table in Appendix A. The mean and the standard deviation for a binomial population are given by:

$$\mu = np \qquad \sigma = \sqrt{pqn}$$

so using the formula

$$z = \frac{X - \mu}{\sigma} \tag{9-5}$$

we should be able to compute a z score that we can use to enter Appendix A with and find the "area smaller" in column #4. For our data:

$$\mu = \tfrac{1}{2}(10) = 5.0 \qquad \sigma = \sqrt{(\tfrac{1}{2})(\tfrac{1}{2})(10)} = 1.58$$

and substituting these values into formula 9.5 with $X = 8$ for the eight female infants we have:

$$z = \frac{8 - 5}{1.58} = 1.90$$

Looking up $z = 1.90$ in Appendix A gives us a probability of 0.0287 which is close to the value obtained using permutations and the binomial theorem (0.0547). The reason that the value obtained using z scores does not equal the value obtained using the other methods is that we are dealing with discrete data and using a table based upon a continuous variable to evaluate these data. In order to correct for this fact, we should use a correction for continuity as follows:

$$z = \frac{|X - \mu| - .5}{\sigma} = \frac{|8 - 5| - .5}{1.58} = 1.58 \tag{9-6}$$

A z score of 1.58 cuts off an area of 0.0571 which is much closer to the value of 0.0547 obtained when we computed the probability directly. Since the z score method is an approximation, it should only be used when np and nq are both equal to five or more.

In summary, we can determine the probability of the outcome of a binomial experiment in four ways. We can do this by listing all the possible outcomes if there are not too many of them; we can use permutations; we can use the binomial theorem; and we can use *z* scores if np and nq are both greater than or equal to 5.

After we have determined the probability of the outcome of our experiment, we must use this information to arrive at a decision. In our example we found that the probability of 8 or more female infants in 10 births is 0.0547. This means that out of every 100 samples of 10 live births each, we would expect about 5 of these 100 to contain 8 or more girls. As an experimenter you must decide if this event occurs so infrequently when only chance is operating that you believe that in this case the result was due to the pill and not to chance. Typically, if the event would happen less than 5 times in 100 ($p \leq .05$) or less than 1 time in 100 ($p \leq .01$) by chance alone, the experimenter concludes that something other than chance is operating. Since we would expect 8 or more females to occur slightly more often than 5 times in 100, we would conclude in this case that the birth-control pill did not affect the sex of the child ($p \leq .05$).

Chapter 10

Testing Hypotheses About Means

Any set of scores may be converted to z scores having reference to a distribution with a mean of zero and a standard deviation of one by use of the formula:

$$z = \frac{X - \mu}{\sigma} \qquad (10\text{--}1)$$

If the raw scores are normally distributed, then we may use the computed z scores to enter Appendix A. If we do not know μ and/or σ but have drawn a random sample, we may compute $\overline{X}$ and s and substitute these into formula 10.1 for their corresponding parameters. Again we must be able to assume that X is normally distributed before we can use Appendix A.

Difference Between a Sample Mean and a Population Mean

Occasionally we know the population mean and standard deviation and are interested in determining whether a particular sample differs significantly from μ. If the mean and standard deviation of a nationally used nursing school admissions test are 500 and 100, respectively, and the mean and standard deviation of our freshman class on this exam are 517 and 98, respectively ($N = 144$), is our class mean significantly different from the population mean of 500? Again we may use a z score to arrive at a decision. The formula used in this case is:

$$z = \frac{\overline{X} - \mu}{\sigma_{\overline{x}}} \qquad (10\text{--}2)$$

or

$$z = \frac{\overline{X} - \mu}{s_{\overline{x}}} \qquad (10\text{--}3)$$

where $\sigma_{\overline{x}}$ and $s_{\overline{x}}$ are standard errors of the mean for the population and the sample and are defined as:

$$\sigma_{\overline{x}} = \sigma/\sqrt{N} \qquad (10\text{--}4)$$
$$s_{\overline{x}} = s/\sqrt{N} \qquad (10\text{--}5)$$

Note that in formula 10.1, the numerator is a difference score and the denominator is a measure of variability appropriate to that difference score, in other words, σ and s measure how raw scores vary about the mean. The same is true of formulas 10.2 and 10.3; the numerator is a difference score and the denominator is a measure of variability appropriate to that difference score, namely, $s_{\overline{x}}$ and $\sigma_{\overline{x}}$ measure how sample means vary about μ. Hence formulas 10.2 and 10.3 produce z scores referenced to a distribution with a mean of zero and a standard deviation of one. In order to look this z score up in Appendix A, we must also be able to assume that it has a normal distribution. This will be the case if: (1) the raw scores are normally distributed or (2) if $\overline{X}$ is based upon a random sample of 30 or more observations. We can then compute the z score for our data as follows:

$$z = \frac{517 - 500}{98/\sqrt{144}} = 2.08$$

Null Hypothesis

Before we can decide if this difference is significant we need to discuss hypothesis testing. All statistical tests have a null hypothesis, an alternative hypothesis, and an alpha level associated with them. The **null hypothesis,** designated H_0, is a statement that a difference does not exist. The **alternative**

hypothesis, designated H_1, is a statement that a difference does exist. The **alpha level,** α, is the probability level chosen by the investigator. If the computed value for z corresponds to a probability smaller than the alpha level selected, then the null hypothesis is rejected in favor of the alternative hypothesis.

Returning to the example of our nursing class exam mean; the null hypothesis would be that the class mean was not different from the population mean; the alternative hypothesis is that the class mean is different from the population mean; we will choose an alpha level of .05.

$$H_0: \overline{X} = \mu$$
$$H_1: \overline{X} \neq \mu$$
$$\alpha = .05$$

The z score we computed using our data was 2.08, and this cuts off an area equal to 0.0188 above it under the normal curve so that the probability of randomly selecting a sample with a mean that differs from μ by 17 points or more is $2(0.0188) = 0.0376$. Since this value is less than our alpha level of .05, we reject H_0 in favor of H_1 and conclude that our sample mean is significantly different from the population mean ($P \leq .05$).

Two-Tailed Tests
Versus One-Tailed Tests

The test that we have just completed is referred to as a two-tailed test of significance. The null hypothesis stated that a true difference did not exist between the population mean and the sample mean, so we took our alpha level and divided it in half between the two tails of the normal distribution. (Rather than always having to look up values in Appendix A, many investigators find it convenient to remember that $z = \pm 1.96$ cuts off an area of 0.025 in each tail of the distribution and thus any computed values of z that exceeds ± 1.96 is significant at $P \leq .05$).

Occasionally the experimenter has reason to predict that if a difference exists it will be in a specific direction. That is, rather than asking whether our class mean differs from the population mean, we could have asked if our class mean was larger than the population mean? The first question tests for the sample mean being smaller or larger than the population mean while the second question looks at the case where the sample mean is larger than the population mean. The second question results in a one-tailed test with the following hypotheses:

$$H_0: \overline{X} \le \mu$$
$$H_1: \overline{X} > \mu$$
$$\alpha = .05$$

When we use a one-tailed test of significance we do not split alpha between the two tails of the distribution but keep it all in one tail. Looking up .05 in column #4 of Appendix A we see that this corresponds to $z = 1.64$, so that if our computed value for z exceeds 1.64, we would reject the null hypothesis. You will notice that for a given alpha level, the table value that we must exceed in order to reject the null hypothesis is smaller for a one-tailed test than for a two-tailed test. The decision to use a one-tailed test should be made a priori, that is, before the investigator has collected any data. Likewise the choice of alpha should be made beforehand.

Difference Between Two Sample Means—Independent Data (N ≥ 30)

Dr. L wants to evaluate two diets, so she randomly divides 60 dieters into two groups, assigns each group a diet, and records the weight lost by each patient during a four-week period with the results recorded in Table 10.1.

Table 10.1. *Weight lost by individuals on two diets*

Diet A				Diet B	
6	8	11	14	9	11
13	7	10	10	16	16
12	13	9	15	12	14
10	10	10	17	13	14
14	11	10	12	15	12
9	9	12	13	13	13
8	12	10	13	15	11
10	8	11	13	11	13
11	9	7	12	14	12
9	11	10	13	10	14

The mean weight lost by patients on diet A is 10.0 pounds and by patients on diet B 13.0 pounds. The question that now confronts Dr. L is, "Is a mean of 13 significantly different from a mean of 10?"

$$H_0: \mu_1 = \mu_2$$
$$H_1: \mu_1 \neq \mu_2$$
$$\alpha = .05$$

This question can also be answered by use of the z statistic. In the numerator we will have the difference between the two means and in the denominator will be a measure of variability appropriate to the numerator, the **standard error of the difference between means,** $s_{\bar{x}_1 - \bar{x}_2}$

$$z = \frac{\bar{X}_1 - \bar{X}_2}{s_{\bar{x}_1 - \bar{x}_2}} \tag{10-6}$$

where:

$$s_{\bar{x}_1 - \bar{x}_2} = \sqrt{\frac{\Sigma X_1^2 - (\Sigma X_1)^2/N_1}{N_1(N_1 - 1)} + \frac{\Sigma X_2^2 - (\Sigma X_2)^2/N_2}{N_2(N_2 - 1)}} \tag{10-7}$$

Substituting the data in Table 10.1 into formula 10.7, we have:

$$z = \frac{13 - 10}{\sqrt{\dfrac{5172 - (390)^2/30}{30(30 - 1)} + \dfrac{3102 - (300)^2/30}{30(30 - 1)}}} = 6.25$$

Since our computed value for z is greater than the table value ($6.25 > \pm 1.96$), Dr. L should reject the null hypothesis and conclude that the diets do produce different results.

Differences Between Two Sample Means—Correlated Data ($N \geq 30$)

In the preceding example our investigator had 60 patients that she assigned to two different groups so that she had two means based upon two independent sets of scores. If the subjects in the two groups are matched with regard to a variable before the start of the project or if the same individuals are measured twice, we are dealing with correlated data rather than independent data. This situation may be analyzed using the formula:

$$z = \frac{\overline{D}}{\sqrt{\dfrac{\Sigma D^2 - (\Sigma D)^2/N}{N(N - 1)}}} \tag{10-8}$$

where D is the difference between each pair of scores.

Table 10.2. *Diastolic blood pressure (mm Hg) before and after treatment with reserpine*

Before	After	D	Before	After	D	Before	After	D
96	86	10	107	96	11	127	109	18
119	103	16	118	104	14	116	103	13
108	92	16	97	87	10	99	89	10
119	107	12	124	108	16	104	93	11
126	110	16	117	103	14	122	106	16
110	98	12	111	100	11	109	100	9
128	107	21	114	102	12	105	94	11
95	86	9	120	105	15	115	103	12
125	109	16	100	91	9	102	92	10
112	110	12	123	108	15	103	92	11
	$\Sigma D = 388$		$\Sigma D^2 = 5280$		$N = 30$	$\overline{D} = 12.9$		

Dr. P measured the diastolic blood pressure on each of 30 patients, gave each patient an injection of reserpine, and measured blood pressure again after an appropriate interval. The data are recorded in Table 10.2.

$$H_0: \mu_B = \mu_A$$
$$H_1: \mu_B \neq \mu_A$$
$$\alpha = .01$$

$$z = \frac{12.9}{\sqrt{\dfrac{5280 - (388)^2/30}{30(29)}}} = 23.45$$

Since 23.45 is greater than the table value of 2.58, H_0 is rejected.

As stated previously, to make use of Appendix A we must have scores that are normally distributed. If we are considering how one score differs from the mean (formula 10.1), we have to be able to assume that X is normally distributed. If we are asking if a sample mean differs from a population mean (formula 10.2 or 10.3) or if two sample means differ from each other (formulas 10.6 or 10.8), we indicated that these sample means must be based upon 30 or more observations. This is because of the **central limit theorem** which states:

> If a population distribution of any shape has a mean (μ) and a standard deviation (σ), then the sampling distribution of sample means computed on samples randomly drawn from this population will approach a normal distribution with a mean (μ) and a standard error of σ/N as N increases.

When $N \geq 30$ this approximation to a normal distribution is usually sufficient to use Appendix A.

t Tests ($N < 30$)

If we wish to test the null hypothesis that two means are different and we have samples smaller than 30, we use a *t* test. If we have two independent samples the formula for *t* is:

$$t = \frac{\overline{X}_1 - \overline{X}_2}{\sqrt{\frac{\Sigma X_1^2 - (\Sigma X_1)^2/N_1 + \Sigma X_2^2 - (\Sigma X_2)^2/N_2}{N_1 + N_2 - 2}\left[\frac{1}{N_1} + \frac{1}{N_2}\right]}} \quad (10\text{–}9)$$

In the case of repeated measures on the same group of subjects, the formula for *t* is the same as that used for *z* in this situation:

$$t = \frac{\overline{D}}{\sqrt{\frac{\Sigma D^2 - (\Sigma D)^2/N}{N(N - 1)}}} \quad (10\text{–}10)$$

The formulas for *z* and *t* are very similar, and they may be used to evaluate the same null hypotheses about means. The main difference between the two statistics is in the tables used to evaluate them. A *z* score is evaluated using Appendix A, and for a given alpha level the cut-off value found in the table is always the same, for example, $\alpha = .05$ yields $z = \pm 1.96$. The *t* test is evaluated using Appendix B, and for a given alpha level the cut-off value in this table changes with each change in sample size. Appendix B is entered using **degrees of freedom,** *df*. The degrees of freedom for two independent samples are: $df = N_1 + N_2 - 2$. If we had a situation where our two means were based upon samples of size 10 and 18, then we would enter the first column in Appendix B and go down it until we find $df = 10 + 18 - 2 = 26$ and then read across this row. For a two-tailed test, $\alpha = .05$, $df = 26$, we find that the table value for the *t* test is 2.056; so if our computed value for *t* exceeded 2.056, we would reject the null hypothesis.

In the case where we have repeated measures on the same subjects, the degrees of freedom for the *t* test are: $df = N - 1$.

Assumptions for *t* Tests

Since $N < 30$ when we use the *t* test, the central limit theorem does not hold and we must be able to assume that our samples are randomly drawn from normal distributions. Furthermore, we must be able to assume that the variances of the two groups are equal, that is, that we have **homogeneity of variances.** The assumption of homogeneity of variances may itself be tested statistically by use of an *F* test which is considered in Chapter 12. If we do not have homogeneity of variances, the *t* test may still be used but the table values for *t* found in Appendix B are no longer appropriate. A new table must be generated using the formula (for $\alpha = .05$):

$$t_{.05} = \frac{s_{\bar{x}_1}^2 (t_1) + s_{\bar{x}_2}^2 (t_2)}{s_{\bar{x}_1}^2 + s_{\bar{x}_2}^2} \qquad (10\text{--}11)$$

where:

$$t_1 = \text{Appendix B value for } \alpha = .05, \, df = N_1 - 1$$
$$t_2 = \text{Appendix B value for } \alpha = .05, \, df = N_2 - 1$$

Errors

Having stated that we do not prove things absolutely in statistics and that all conclusions are made at a particular alpha level, let us investigate this matter in a little more detail. Consider the case of the investigator who has developed a new, cheap screening test for cancer. This test cost 35¢ to mass-produce, can be self-administered at home, and the investigator has a company that is interested in manufacturing it. He has given the test to 10,000 people who have been diagnosed by other means as having cancer and to 10,000 people who are, as far as he can tell, cancer-free. The two distributions are normal, and the means and standard deviations are:

$$\mu_{NC} = 100 \qquad \sigma_{NC} = 10 \qquad \mu_C = 122 \qquad \sigma_C = 5$$

Our investigator now wishes to write out the instructions for his test and include a statement saying, "If your score exceeds *Y*, there is a chance that you may have cancer, and so you should make an appointment with your physician as soon as possible for a physical exam." His problem is what number to put in the instructions for "*Y*." If we write this in terms of a null hypothesis, we have:

$$H_0: Y \leq \mu_{NC}$$
$$H_1: Y > \mu_{NC}$$

that is, the person's score is from the noncancer population. (Since the cancer population falls above the noncancer population on this test, we have chosen to use a one-tailed test.) Suppose that our investigator decides on an alpha level of .05. A z equal to 1.64 cuts off 5% of the area of the normal curve above it, so substituting into formula 10.1 we have:

$$1.64 = \frac{Y - 100}{10}$$

$$Y = 116.4$$

Therefore, he should replace Y with 116.4 in his instructions.

Note that 5% of the time people who do not have cancer will have test scores of 116.4 or higher. For these people he has made an error: he has rejected the null hypothesis when the null hypothesis was in fact true. This is referred to as a **Type I error,** and the probability of making it is given by alpha. We can also see from Figure 10.1 that some of the people who have cancer will have test scores below 116.4. For these individuals he will also make an error: he will accept the null hypothesis when in fact he should have rejected it. This is called a **Type II error,** and its probability is given by beta. In this case beta is the area under the cancer curve below a value of 116.4. We can determine beta numerically using formula 10.1:

$$z = \frac{116.4 - 122}{5} = -1.12$$

A z of -1.12 cuts off an area of 0.13 below it; so $\beta = .13$.

If the investigator decided that an alpha of .05 was too low and changed to an alpha level of .01, he would reduce the probability of making a Type I error but at the same time he would increase the probability of making a Type II error. These two types of error are not independent, so the investigator must decide which type of error is more expensive to make in the given situation.

The **power** of a statistical test is the probability of rejecting the null hypothesis when the null hypothesis is false. Numerically it is equal to one minus beta:

$$\text{Power} = 1 - \beta \qquad (10\text{--}12)$$

or, for our example:

$$\text{Power} = 1 - .13 = .87$$

If we have a choice between two statistical tests to test a particular null hypothesis, we should choose the one with the greater power.

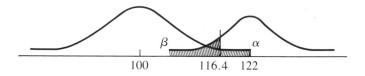

100   116.4 122

Figure 10.1.   *The relationship between Type I and Type II error*

Exercise 10

1. Hemoglobin levels (g/100 ml) were measured on 16 normal males and 14 normal females. Determine if there is a difference in the mean hemoglobin level between the sexes.

Males		Females	
14.7	16.1	13.5	14.5
13.8	13.4	13.9	12.9
13.7	14.9	13.2	14.3
14.8	16.1	14.4	13.6
15.2	13.1	14.6	13.5
15.4	16.4	13.2	13.8
15.5	13.0	13.7	12.5
15.7	14.4		

2. In order to evaluate the effect of elevation upon blood pressure, an investigator measured systolic blood pressure (mm Hg) of ten hypertensive patients after they had been sitting in a chair for ten minutes and again after they had been lying prone for ten minutes. Determine if the position of the patient affected the blood pressure measurements.

Patient #	Sitting	Prone
1	210	185
2	170	175
3	160	155
4	180	170
5	190	190
6	200	195
7	160	165
8	170	172
9	190	185
10	180	185

3. You have developed a new IQ test to be used in screening mentally re-tarded children. You have given this test to 10,000 "normals" and to 4,000 children diagnosed as being mentally retarded. The resulting parameters are:

$$\mu_n = 100; \ \sigma_n = 15 \qquad \mu_{mr} = 80; \ \sigma_{mr} = 20$$

(a) Determine the IQ score below which 5% of the normal children will fall.

(b) Using the value found in (a) as the cut-off point for normals, find the probability of making a Type II error.

(c) What is the power of this test?

Chapter 11

Testing Hypotheses About Correlations

H_0: $r = 0$; $N \geq 30$

Having once computed Pearson's r for a set of data, we may want to know if this value is statistically significant. Suppose that you have a computed value of $r = .23$ based upon 101 pairs of scores and you would like to test the hypothesis:

$$H_0: r = 0$$

$$H_1: r \neq 0$$

$$\alpha = .05$$

This can be accomplished with the z statistics. The standard error of r is:

$$s_r = 1/\sqrt{N - 1} \qquad (11\text{--}1)$$

so that z is defined in this case as:

$$z = \frac{r}{1/\sqrt{N - 1}} = r(\sqrt{N - 1}) \qquad (11\text{--}2)$$

For your data we have:

$$z = .23(\sqrt{101 - 1}) = 2.30$$

Since the computed value for z exceeds the table value in Appendix A for the chosen alpha level ($2.30 > \pm 1.96$), you reject the null hypothesis and conclude that your correlation is significantly different from zero.

H_0: $r = 0$; $N < 30$

If the correlation coefficient is based upon less than 30 pairs of scores, we must use a t test to test this null hypothesis. In order to evaluate a value of $r = .94$ based upon four pairs of observations, we would use the formula:

$$t = \frac{r\sqrt{N-2}}{\sqrt{1-r^2}} \qquad \text{with } df = N - 2 \qquad (11\text{--}3)$$

so we have:

$$t = \frac{.94\sqrt{2}}{\sqrt{1 - .94^2}} = 3.87$$

Entering Appendix B with $df = 4 - 2 = 2$, we obtain a table value of ± 4.30 corresponding to $\alpha = .05$. Since $3.87 < \pm 4.30$, we must accept the null hypothesis of no difference.

The reader should compare these two examples and note that sample size is a crucial factor in determining if r equals 0. Small values of r may differ significantly from zero if they are based upon a large number of observations, while large values of r may not differ from zero if they are based upon a small number of observations. It is for this reason that the **coefficient of determination,** r^2, is useful if one is contemplating the use of regression. The coefficient of determination tells us how much of the variation in Y is predictable on the basis of variation in X. In our first example, $r = .23$ did differ significantly from zero, but r^2 equals .05 so that the amount of variation that is predictable is so small that regression would not be of practical use even though r is significant.

H_0: $\rho = 0$

The Spearman rank order correlation coefficient may be tested by substituting ρ for r in the t test formula 11.3. If $N \le 10$, special tables are available to evaluate ρ (Edwards, 1967, p. 437).

$H_0: r_{pb} = 0$

The point biserial correlation coefficient is also tested by replacing r in formula 11.3 with r_{pb}.

$H_0: r_b = 0$

The biserial correlation coefficient is tested using the formula:

$$t = \frac{(r_b)(y\ \sqrt{N})}{\sqrt{pq}} \tag{11-4}$$

with $df = N - 2$.

$H_0: \phi = 0$

The phi coefficient is tested using the chi square statistic discussed in Chapter 13.

$$\chi^2 = N\phi^2 \tag{11-5}$$

with $df = 1$.

$H_0: \eta = 0$

The curvilinear correlation, eta, is tested using the F statistic covered in Chapter 12.

$$F = \frac{SS_{between\ columns}/(k-1)}{SS_{within\ columns}/(N-k)} \tag{11-6}$$

with $df = (k - 1), (N - k)$.

$H_0: r_1 = r_2$

Independent Data

If the correlation between two variables in the population is zero, then the sampling distribution of r will be normal with a mean of zero. On the other hand, if $r \neq 0$ in the population, then the sampling distribution of r will not be normal since r has upper and lower limits which it can not exceed (± 1).

The larger the true value for r is, the more skewed will be its sampling distribution. Since the sampling distribution for r is not normal in this case, the sampling distribution of the differences between two r's will not be normal either. For this reason the values of the correlation coefficients can not be put directly into a z formula but must be transformed into scores that are normally distributed. Fisher's z' transformation transforms r into z' which is normally distributed. Appendix H lists various values of r in the body of the table and their corresponding z' values on the margin.

The standard error of the difference between two independent z's is:

$$s_{z'_1 - z'_2} = \sqrt{\frac{1}{N_1 - 3} + \frac{1}{N_2 - 3}} \tag{11-7}$$

and hence:

$$z = \frac{z'_1 - z'_2}{\sqrt{\dfrac{1}{N_1 - 3} + \dfrac{1}{N_2 - 3}}} \tag{11-8}$$

Consider the case of the researcher who has replicated an experiment and has obtained two Pearson's r's:

$$r_1 = .72; \; N_1 = 28 \qquad r_2 = .60; \; N_2 = 53$$

She would like to pool the data from these two replications but is concerned that they might be different; so she wishes to test the hypothesis:

$$H_0\!: r_1 = r_2$$
$$H_1\!: r_1 \neq r_2$$
$$\alpha = .05$$

Looking up correlations of .71 and .60 in Appendix H, we find that these correspond to z' values of .91 and .69, respectively. Substituting these values into formula 11.8 we have:

$$z = \frac{.91 - .69}{\sqrt{\dfrac{1}{28 - 3} + \dfrac{1}{53 - 3}}} = .88$$

Since $.88 < \pm 1.96$, our researcher accepts the null hypothesis of no difference and can pool her data.

Correlated Data

If we have two correlations that are not independent, then the preceding z score may not be used. Suppose that we have computed correlations between height and weight (r_{xy}) and between height and blood pressure (r_{xz}) on 25 patients. We want to know if these two correlations are significantly different. In this case the formula to use is:

$$t = \frac{(r_{xy} - r_{xz})\ \sqrt{(N-3)(1 + r_{yz})}}{\sqrt{2(1 - r_{xy}^2 - r_{xz}^2 - r_{yz}^2 + 2r_{xy}r_{xz}r_{yz})}} \qquad \text{with } df = N - 3 \qquad (11\text{–}9)$$

$H_0: b_y = 0$

It can be shown that testing the hypothesis that the regression coefficient is equal to zero is equivalent to testing the hypothesis that r equals 0. This has already been discussed.

$H_0: b_{y_1} = b_{y_2}$

If we wish to determine if the slopes of two regression lines, based upon independent data, differ significantly from each other, we must first compute the pooled standard error of estimate using formula 11.10:

$$s_{b_y} = \sqrt{\frac{\left(\Sigma Y_1^2 - \frac{(\Sigma Y_1)^2}{N_1}\right) - \frac{\left(\Sigma X_1 Y_1 - \frac{(\Sigma X_1)(\Sigma Y_1)}{N_1}\right)^2}{\Sigma X_1^2 - \frac{(\Sigma X_1)^2}{N_1}} + \left(\Sigma Y_2^2 - \frac{(\Sigma Y_2)^2}{N_2}\right) - \frac{\left(\Sigma X_2 Y_2 - \frac{(\Sigma X_2)(\Sigma Y_2)}{N_2}\right)^2}{\Sigma X_2^2 - \frac{(\Sigma X_2)^2}{N_2}}}{N_1 + N_2 - 4}} \qquad (11\text{–}10)$$

The s_{b_y} is used to compute the standard error of the difference between two regression coefficients, $s_{b_y - b_y}$

$$s_{b_{y_1} - b_{y_2}} = \sqrt{s_{b_y}^2 \left(\frac{1}{\Sigma X_1^2 - \frac{(\Sigma X_1)^2}{N_1}} + \frac{1}{\Sigma X_2^2 - \frac{(\Sigma X_2)^2}{N_2}}\right)} \qquad (11\text{–}11)$$

This standard error is used as the denominator of a t test, formula 11.12, with $df = N_1 + N_2 - 4$:

$$t = \frac{b_{y_1} - b_{y_2}}{s_{b_{y_1} - b_{y_2}}} \qquad (11\text{–}12)$$

Exercise 11

Test the following null hypothesis:

1. H_0: $r = 0$ $N = 39$ $r = .58$
2. H_0: $\rho = 0$ $N = 23$ $\rho = .68$
3. H_0: $r_b = 0$ $N = 25$ $r_b = .50$ $p = .6$
4. H_0: $\phi = 0$ $N = 100$ $\phi = .21$
5. H_0: $r_1 = r_2$ $N_1 = 28$ $r_1 = .811$ (independent)
                        $N_2 = 23$ $r_2 = .917$

Chapter 12

F Test and the Analysis of Variance

The *F* statistic is defined as the ratio of two variances, and it is used to compare variances. It may be used to test the assumption of homogeneity of variances for the *t* test and, more important, it is the basis of the analysis of variance

F Test

Dr. M has two independent groups and she plans to do a *t* test to see if their means differ. The variances and *N*'s for the two groups are:

$$s_1^2 = 15.1; \ N_1 = 8 \qquad s_2^2 = 3.2; \ N_2 = 10$$

Inspection of these data leads her to suspect that she does not have homogeneity of variances, and so she wishes to test the null hypothesis:

$$H_0: \sigma_1^2 = \sigma_2^2$$
$$H_1: \sigma_1^2 \neq \sigma_2^2$$
$$\alpha = .01$$

In this situation the F statistic is defined as the ratio of the larger variance to the smaller:

$$F = s^2_{\text{larger}}/s^2_{\text{smaller}}$$

For Dr. M's data we have $F = 15.1/3.2 = 4.72$. The F statistic is evaluated by using Appendix C. Like the t test, we need degrees of freedom to enter this table. The degrees of freedom for the numerator of the F ratio are the number of observations that the numerator is based upon minus one ($df_n = 8 - 1 = 7$); the degrees of freedom for the denominator are equal to the number of observations that the denominator is based upon minus one ($df_d = 10 - 1 = 9$). To find the critical value for F we go across the top of Appendix C to the df's for the numerator and down the side of the table to the df's for the denominator; the intersection of this column and row contains the critical values. In our example we have $df = 7,9$ and the table value for $\alpha = .01$ is 5.61. The interpretation of F is identical to z or the t test, that is, if the computed value for F exceeds the table value for the chosen alpha level, we reject the null hypothesis. Since Dr. M computed a value of 4.72 for F and the table value is 5.61, she would accept the null hypothesis and conclude that the assumption of homogeneity has been satisfied.

Analysis of Variance

The analysis of variance, ANOVA, is used to test for differences between means when we have three or more groups. If the number of groups is small, this could be done by using t tests, but as the number of groups increases, this procedure becomes prohibitive. Additionally, the ANOVA allows us to statistically evaluate interaction terms that are not directly accessible when we use t tests.

The ANOVA is based on the same underlying assumptions as the z and t statistics. We must have random samples, and if the N's are less than 30, we must be able to assume that we have normal distributions and homogeneity of variances in the groups.

The final test in the ANOVA is an F test which is, as we have already seen, a statistic composed of the ratio of two variances. Thus we are going to use a statistic based upon variances to test a null hypothesis about means, namely, $\mu_1 = \mu_2 = \mu_3 \cdot \cdot \cdot \mu_k$. Let us begin by defining some terms commonly encountered in the ANOVA. s^2 is a variance and if we look at its theoretical formula, we have:

$$s^2 = \frac{\Sigma(X - \overline{X})^2}{N - 1} \tag{12--2}$$

The numerator is the "sum of the squared deviations about the mean" and in ANOVA language this is shortened to the "sum of squares" or abbreviated "SS." The denominator is the degrees of freedom associated with the numerator. A variance is referred to as a "Mean Square" or "MS," so the F statistic in an ANOVA is the ratio of two MS's:

$$F = \frac{MS_1}{MS_2} \qquad (12\text{--}3)$$

where:

$$MS = \frac{SS}{df} \qquad (12\text{--}4)$$

One reason for breaking a MS into a SS and corresponding df's is that SS's are additive, df's are additive, but MS's are not.

Single Classification ANOVA — Independent Data

Consider the experiment where 15 rats have been randomly assigned to one of three groups, each group is injected with a different dosage of a drug, and serum levels of the drug are measured four hours later. Do these dosages produce different mean serum levels?

$$H_0: \mu_1 = \mu_2 = \mu_3$$
$$H_1: H_0 \text{ is false}$$
$$\alpha = .05$$

In order to simplify things, let us begin by considering only the *sums of squares* and defining the following terms:

$k =$ the number of groups

$n =$ the number of observations per group

$N = kn =$ the total number of observations in the experiment

$X_{ij} =$ the observation in row i, column j of the data matrix

$\bar{T}_j = \Sigma X_j / n_j =$ the mean of observations made under treatment j

$G = \Sigma X_{ij} =$ the sum of all kn observations

$\bar{G} = \Sigma X_{ij} / N =$ the mean of all the observations in the experiment

If we ignore the fact that animals have been assigned to different groups, we can compute a *total sums of squares* by determining how each score differs from the grand mean of all kn observations, squaring these differences and summing.

$$SS_{total} = \Sigma (X_{ij} - \bar{G})^2 \qquad (12\text{--}5)$$

We can also compute the variability within each group by determining how the scores in that group vary about that group mean. If we do this for each group and then sum these values, we will have the *sums of squares within groups:*

$$SS_{within} = \Sigma\Sigma(X_{ij} - \overline{T}_j)^2$$
$$= \Sigma(X_{i1} - \overline{T}_1)^2 + \Sigma(X_{i2} - \overline{T}_2)^2 + \cdots + \Sigma(X_{ik} - \overline{T}_k)^2 \quad (12\text{–}6)$$

We may also complete the *sum of squares between groups* by considering how each group mean varies about the grand mean.

$$SS_{between} = n\Sigma(\overline{T}_j - \overline{G})^2 \quad (12\text{–}7)$$

Formulas 12.5, 12.6, and 12.7 allow us to see what each of these SS's is measuring, but they are very cumbersome to use in actual computations. To compute these three values we will find the following formulas more convenient to use in most situations:

$$SS_{total} = \Sigma X_{ij}^2 - \frac{G^2}{N} \quad (12\text{–}8)$$

$$SS_{between} = \frac{\Sigma T_j^2}{n_j} - \frac{G^2}{N} \quad (12\text{–}9)$$

$$SS_{within} = \Sigma X_{ij}^2 - \frac{\Sigma T_j^2}{n_j} \quad (12\text{–}10)$$

After we have computed these SS's, we can divide each by its degrees of freedom to produce the corresponding MS. The total number of degrees of freedom is equal to the total number of observations minus one:

$$df_{total} = N - 1$$

The degrees of freedom within is equal to the number of degrees of freedom in each group times the number of groups. The degrees of freedom between groups is equal to the number of groups minus one:

$$df_{within} = k(n - 1)$$
$$df_{between} = k - 1$$

Once we have computed these values, we have a check on our computations because degrees of freedom and sums of squares are additive:

$$SS_{total} = SS_{within} + SS_{between}$$
$$df_{total} = df_{within} + df_{between}$$

The final F ratio for this type of design is composed of the $MS_{between}$ divided by the MS_{within}.

Table 12.1. *Raw data for single classification ANOVA*

5 mg	10 mg	15 mg	
4	5	5	$k = 3$
2	2	4	$n = 5$
1	3	3	$G = 48$
3	3	5	
1	3	4	
11	16	21	

Now let us assume that or experiment has produced the data in Table 12.1 for our three groups of rats.

$$\Sigma X_{ij}^2 = 4^2 + 2^2 + 1^2 + \cdots + 5^2 + 4^2 = 178$$

$$\frac{\Sigma T_j^2}{n_j} = \frac{11^2 + 16^2 + 21^2}{5} = 163.6$$

$$\frac{G^2}{N} = \frac{48^2}{15} = 153.6$$

Substituting these values into formula 12.8 we can determine the SS_{total}:

$$SS_{total} = 178 - 153.6 = 24.4$$

Likewise $SS_{between}$ and SS_{within} are:

$$SS_{between} = 163.6 - 153.6 = 10.0$$

$$SS_{within} = 178 - 163.6 = 14.4$$

The respective degrees of freedom are:

$$df_{total} = N - 1 + 15 - 1 = 14$$

$$df_{between} = k - 1 = 3 - 1 = 2$$

$$df_{within} = k(n - 1) = 3(5 - 1) = 12$$

The $MS_{between} = 10/2 = 5.0$ and the $MS_{within} = 14.4/12 = 1.2$, so $F = 5.0/1.2 = 4.17$ with 2 and 12 degrees of freedom. Entering Appendix C with 2 and 12 degrees of freedom we see that our value for F exceeds the table value for alpha of .05, so we reject the null hypothesis.

It is customary to report the results of an ANOVA in a summary table with the format shown in Table 12.2. This table shows all the individual sums of

Table 12.2.   *Summary table for single classification ANOVA*

Source	SS	df	MS	F
Total	24.4	14		
Between	10.0	2	5.0	4.17*
Within	14.4	12	1.2	

*Significant at $\alpha = .05$

squares and degrees of freedom. Since the mean squares are not additive, only those of interest are computed and entered in the table. One asterisk denotes significance at the .05 level, two at the .01, and three at .001.

If the ANOVA is significant, we will usually want to investigate the various combinations of treatment means. Several statistical procedures have been developed to make all possible comparisons between individual pairs of means. The one outlined here is called the Scheffé test. It consists of computing an F statistic for each comparison using the formula:

$$F = \frac{(\overline{X}_1 - \overline{X}_2)^2}{MS_\epsilon(n_1 + n_2)/n_1 n_2} \qquad (12\text{--}11)$$

where MS_ϵ is the denominator of the original F test in the ANOVA.

Continuing with our example, to find out if $\overline{X}_1 = \overline{X}_3$ we have:

$$F = \frac{(2.2 - 4.2)^2}{1.2(5 + 5)/(5)(5)} = 8.33*$$

for $\overline{X}_1 = \overline{X}_2$, we have:

$$F = \frac{(2.2 - 3.2)^2}{1.2(5 + 5)/(5)(5)} = 2.08$$

and for $\overline{X}_2 = \overline{X}_3$:

$$F = \frac{(3.2 - 4.2)^2}{1.2(5 + 5)/(5)(5)} = 2.08$$

In order to obtain the critical value used to evaluate these three Scheffé F's, we multiply $(k - 1)$ by the critical value from Appendix C used to evaluate the original F in the ANOVA. For $\alpha = .05$, $df = (2.12)$, Appendix C yields 3.88, so if either of our Scheffé F's exceeds $(3.88)(2) = 7.76$, we would reject the corresponding null hypothesis. In this case, because 2.08 is less than 7.76 we would conclude that $\overline{X}_2$ does not differ from either $\overline{X}_1$ or $\overline{X}_3$.

Single Classification ANOVA—Correlated Data

In the preceding example each group was composed of different individuals—independent data. Like the z and t tests, the ANOVA may also be used when we have correlated data or repeated measurements on the same subjects. In this case the SS_{total} is broken down into $SS_{between\ subjects}$ and $SS_{within\ subjects}$ and then the $SS_{within\ subjects}$ is further fractionated into $SS_{treatments}$ and SS_{error}. The theoretical and computational formulas for these sums of squares are:

$$SS_{total} = \Sigma(X_{ij} - \overline{G})^2 = \Sigma X_{ij}^2 - \frac{G^2}{N} \qquad (12\text{–}12)$$

$$SS_{bet.\ subj.} = k\Sigma(\overline{P}_i - \overline{G})^2 = \frac{\Sigma P_i^2}{k} - \frac{G^2}{N} \qquad (12\text{–}13)$$

$$SS_{within\ subj.} = \Sigma\Sigma(X_{ij} - \overline{P}_i)^2 = \Sigma X_{ij}^2 - \frac{\Sigma P_i^2}{k} \qquad (12\text{–}14)$$

$$SS_{treatment} = n\Sigma(\overline{T}_j - \overline{G})^2 = \frac{\Sigma T_j^2}{n_j} - \frac{G^2}{N} \qquad (12\text{–}15)$$

$$SS_{error} = \Sigma\Sigma[(X_{ij} - \overline{G}) - (\overline{P}_i - \overline{G}) - (\overline{T}_j - \overline{G})]^2$$

$$= \Sigma X_{ij}^2 - \frac{\Sigma T_j^2}{n_j} - \frac{\Sigma P_i^2}{k} + \frac{G^2}{N} \qquad (12\text{–}16)$$

k is still the number of columns in the data matrix, but now it refers to the number of treatment conditions rather than the number of groups. P_i is the sum of all observations made on subject #i, the sum of row i.

As an example, suppose an investigator injects five rats with a compound and then takes blood samples from each of the animals one hour, three hours, and five hours after the injection. He determines the serum level of the compound and records the results in Table 12.3.

Table 12.3. *Raw data for single classification, repeated measures, ANOVA*

Subject	1 Hour	3 Hours	5 Hours	Total
1	5	5	4	14
2	4	2	2	8
3	3	3	1	7
4	5	3	3	11
5	4	3	1	8
	21	16	11	48

$$\frac{G^2}{N} = \frac{48^2}{15} = 153.6$$

$$\Sigma X_{ij}^2 = 5^2 + 4^2 + \cdots + 3^2 + 1^2 = 178$$

$$\frac{\Sigma T_j^2}{n_j} = \frac{21^2 + 16^2 + 11^2}{5} = 163.6$$

$$\frac{\Sigma P_i^2}{k} = \frac{14^2 + 8^2 + 7^2 + 11^2 + 8^2}{3} = 164.7$$

Our sums of squares and their respective degrees of freedom are:

$$SS_{\text{total}} = 178 - 153.6 = 24.4$$

$$SS_{\text{bet. subj.}} = 164.7 - 153.6 = 11.1$$

$$SS_{\text{within subj.}} = 178 - 164.7 = 13.3$$

$$SS_{\text{treatment}} = 163.6 - 153.6 = 10.0$$

$$SS_{\text{error}} = 178 - 163.6 - 164.7 + 153.6 = 3.3$$

$$df_{\text{total}} = N - 1 = 14$$

$$df_{\text{bet. subj.}} = n - 1 = 4$$

$$df_{\text{within subj.}} = n(k - 1) = 10$$

$$df_{\text{treatments}} = k - 1 = 2$$

$$df_{\text{error}} = (n - 1)(k - 1) = 8$$

Sums of squares and degrees of freedom are additive, so we can check our work:

$$SS_{\text{total}} = SS_{\text{bet. subj.}} + SS_{\text{within subj.}} \qquad 24.4 = 11.1 + 13.3$$

$$SS_{\text{within subj.}} = SS_{\text{treatments}} + SS_{\text{error}} \qquad 13.3 = 10.0 + 3.3$$

For this type of design, the F test to determine whether or not the treatment means differ is the ratio of $MS_{\text{treatment}}$ over MS_{error}. Again the work should be reported in a summary table (Table 12.4).

Entering Appendix C with 2 and 8 degrees of freedom, we find that the computed value for F is significant at alpha of .01. Scheffé tests can be made as before on all possible combinations of treatment means.

Table 12.4.   Summary table for single classification, repeated measures, ANOVA

Source	SS	df	MS	F
Total	24.4	14		
Between Subjects	11.1	4		
Within Subjects	13.3	10		
Treatments	10.0	2	5.00	12.19**
Error	3.3	8	.41	

**Significant at $\alpha = .01$

Factorial Experiments

So far we have considered ANOVA schemes that are designed to look at one variable at a time, such as different dosages of a particular drug. ANOVA may also be used in experiments where we wish to consider the effects of two or more variables simultaneously.

Dr. F has conditioned heart rate in two strains of rats. One third of the animals were injected with saline before conditioning, one third with .5 mg/kg of atrophine, and one third with 10 mg/kg atrophine. Fifteen animals were randomly selected from each strain and five were assigned to each drug condition. Heart rate changes were recorded, and the data are listed in Table 12.5. Dr. F wants to know: (1) if there is any difference between the two strains and (2) if there is any difference between the dosages.

In this case we have two variables under study—strain of animal and drug dose. Each variable is present at more than one level. In developing a general notation, let us designate one variable as "factor A" and the other as "factor B." The number of levels of factor A present in the study is designated as p, the number of levels of factor B as q, and there will be n observations in each of the pq cells in the data matrix. In our example we will call the strain variable factor A and the drug variable factor B; then $p = 2$, $q = 3$, and $n = 5$.

Table 12.5.   Raw data for two by three factorial design

	0 mg	.5 mg	10 mg
Strain #1	9, 8, 7, 10, 9	8, 7, 9, 9, 6	0, 3, 1, 4, 2
Strain #2	6, 7, 7, 8, 5	6, 5, 6, 5, 6	1, 0, 0, 1, 1

Table 12.6. *AB summary table for ANOVA*

	B_1	B_2	B_3	
A_1	43	39	10	92
A_2	33	28	3	64
	76	67	13	156

The sum of all observations made under the first level of factor A is designated A_1; the sum of all observations made under the second level of factor A is designated A_2; the sum of all the observations made under the first level of factor B is designated B_1; etc. The sum of all observations made under a given treatment combination is designated AB_{ij}. For example, AB_{12} is the sum of all observations made under the first level of factor A and the second level of factor B. If we sum all the observations in each cell of the raw data matrix, we produce an AB summary table. This table has AB_{ij}'s as cell entries, A_i's as row totals, and B_j's as column totals. For Dr. F's data the AB summary table is found in Table 12.6.

The total variation in this design may be broken down into variation due to factor A, variation due to factor B, variation due to the interaction of factors A and B, and variation due to error:

$$SS_{\text{total}} = SS_A + SS_B + SS_{AB} + SS_\epsilon$$

The computational formulas for these sums of squares are:

$$SS_{\text{total}} = \Sigma X_{ij}^2 - \frac{G^2}{N} \tag{12–17}$$

$$SS_A = \frac{\Sigma A_i^2}{nq} + \frac{G^2}{N} \tag{12–18}$$

$$SS_B = \frac{\Sigma B_j^2}{np} + \frac{G^2}{N} \tag{12–19}$$

$$SS_{AB} = \frac{\Sigma AB_{ij}^2}{n} - \frac{\Sigma A_i^2}{nq} - \frac{\Sigma B_j^2}{np} + \frac{G^2}{N} \tag{12–20}$$

$$SS_\epsilon = \Sigma X_{ij}^2 - \frac{\Sigma AB_{ij}^2}{n} \tag{12–21}$$

Applying these formulas to our example we have:

$$\frac{G^2}{N} = \frac{156^2}{30} = 811.2$$

$$\Sigma X_{ij}^2 = 9^2 + 8^2 + \cdots + 1^2 + 1^2 = 1100$$

$$\frac{\Sigma A_i^2}{nq} = \frac{92^2 + 64^2}{15} = 837.3$$

$$\frac{\Sigma B_j^2}{np} = \frac{76^2 + 67^2 + 13^2}{10} = 1043.4$$

$$\frac{\Sigma A B_{ij}^2}{n} = \frac{43^2 + 39^2 + 10^2 + 33^2 + 28^2 + 3^2}{5} = 1070.4$$

The sums of squares for these data are:

$$SS_{\text{total}} = 1100 - 811.2 = 288.8$$
$$SS_A = 837.3 - 811.2 = 26.1$$
$$SS_B = 1043.4 - 811.2 - 232.2$$
$$SS_{AB} = 1070.4 - 837.3 - 1043.4 + 811.2 = 0.9$$
$$SS_\epsilon = 1100 - 1070.4 = 29.6$$

The corresponding degrees of freedom are:

$$df_{\text{total}} = N - 1 = 30 - 1 = 29$$
$$df_A = p - 1 = 2 - 1 = 1$$
$$df_B = q - 1 = 3 - 1 = 2$$
$$df_{AB} = (P - 1)(q - 1) = (2 - 1)(3 - 1) = 2$$
$$df_\epsilon = pq(n - 1) = 6(5 - 1) = 24$$

The effect of factor A is tested using the F ratio MS_A/MS_ϵ; the effect of factor B is tested by $F = MS_B/MS_\epsilon$; and the interaction is tested with $F = MS_{AB}/MS_\epsilon$. Computing these values and comparing them with Appendix C we find that the interaction with $df = (2, 24)$ is not significant but that factors A and B with $df = (1, 24)$ and $df - (2, 24)$, respectively, are significant at alpha of .01. Dr. *F*'s data may be summarized then in the standard format (Table 12.7).

Since there are only two strains of animals in the experiment, no further analysis of factor A is needed. The significant effect of factor B tells us that

Table 12.7. Summary table for two factor ANOVA

Source	SS	df	MS	F
Total	288.8	29		
Strain	26.1	1	26.10	21.22**
Drug	232.2	2	116.10	94.39**
Strain × Drug	.9	2	.45	.36
Error	29.6	24	1.23	

**Significant at $\alpha = .01$

the saline and 10 mg groups differ; we do not know if the other comparisons are significant too. We can determine this with Scheffé tests as before.

$$H_0: \overline{X}_{\text{saline}} = \overline{X}_{.5\,\text{mg}} \qquad F = \frac{(7.6 - 6.7)^2}{1.23(10 + 10)/100} = 3.24$$

$$H_0: \overline{X}_{.5\,\text{mg}} = \overline{X}_{10\,\text{mg}} \qquad F = \frac{(6.7 - 1.3)^2}{1.23(10 + 10)/100} = 116.6$$

Appendix C gives us a value of 5.61 for alpha of .01 and $df = (2, 24)$, so if either of our Scheffé values exceed $2(5.61) = 11.22$, they are significant. Therefore, we conclude that a dose of 10 mg produces a result significantly different from a dose of .5 mg or from saline but that treatment with saline or .5 mg does not produce a difference.

Interactions

A few brief comments need to be made about interaction terms. An interaction effect will be significant if the combining of the factors produces something unique, such as if the result of the combination can not be predicted from the individual factors. Some people find it easier to understand interactions pictorially, and we have graphed Dr. F's data from the AB summary table in Figure 12.1. Here the two lines are close to being parallel and hence the interaction is not significant. Regardless of the drug dosage, strain #1 always has a higher total.

In order to gain more insight into interaction terms, consider the following example. Dr. M wants to evaluate two methods of teaching reading and wants to study these methods on both "normals" and mentally retarded children. She randomly selects ten normal children and assigns five of them to each method; likewise ten mentally retarded children are selected and assigned. After four months of instruction all 20 children are given the same 25 point test, and the data are given in Tables 12.8 and 12.9.

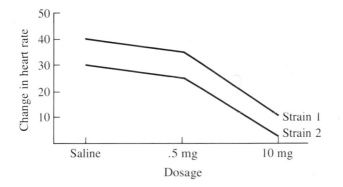

Figure 12.1.   *Group totals from Dr. F's ANOVA*

Table 12.8.   *Raw data for a two by two factorial design*

	Method #1	Method #2
Normals	20, 25, 18, 17, 20	12, 8, 9, 6, 10
MR's	11, 8, 6, 7, 8	20, 17, 20, 18, 20

Table 12.9.   *AB summary table*

	Method #1	Method #2	
Normals	100	45	145
MR's	40	95	135
	140	140	280

Designating "type of pupil" as factor A and "method" as factor B, we proceed with the computations:

$$\frac{G^2}{N} = \frac{280^2}{20} = 3920$$

$$\Sigma X_{ij}^2 = 4610$$

$$\frac{\Sigma A_i^2}{nq} = \frac{145^2 + 135^2}{10} = 3925$$

$$\frac{\Sigma B_j^2}{np} = \frac{140^2 + 140^2}{10} = 3920$$

$$\frac{\Sigma AB_{ij}^2}{n} = \frac{100^2 + 40^2 + 45^2 + 95^2}{5} = 4530$$

$$SS_{total} = 4610 - 3920 = 690 \qquad\qquad df_{total} = 20 - 1 = 19$$

$$SS_A = 3925 - 3920 = 5 \qquad\qquad df_A = 2 - 1 = 1$$

$$SS_B = 3920 - 3920 = 0 \qquad\qquad df_B = 2 - 1 = 1$$

$$SS_{AB} = 4530 - 3925 - 3920 + 3920 = 605 \qquad df_{AB} = (2 - 1)(2 - 1) = 1$$

$$SS_\epsilon = 4610 - 4530 = 80 \qquad\qquad df_\epsilon = 4(5 - 1) = 16$$

As can be seen in Table 12.10, the interaction is significant but the factors are not. However, consider the graph of the summary table in Figure 12.2. Here the lines cross; Method #1 is best for normals but Method #2 is best for MR's. In situations such as this where there is a significant interaction, it may not make sense to look at the individual factors. The significant interaction masks their effects. In this case the ANOVA did not detect a difference between the two methods or between the two types of pupils, but the graph in Figure 12.2 suggests that these differences do exist. A more detailed analysis of simple effects is called for in this case but this is beyond the scope of this text. The reader is referred to Winer (1971) for these procedures.

Whole courses and texts are devoted to ANOVA and its many uses. Our attempt here is only to provide a very brief introduction to some of the more commonly encountered types of designs.

Table 12.10.   *Summary table for two factor ANOVA*

Source	SS	df	MS	F
Total	690	19		
Pupils	5	1	5	1.00
Methods	0	1	0	0.00
Pupils × Methods	605	1	605	121.00**
Error	80	16	5	

**Significant at $\alpha = .01$

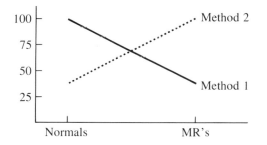

Figure 12.2.   *Diagram of significant ANOVA interaction*

Exercise 12

1. In order to evaluate three diets 18 rats were randomly assigned to one of three groups and each group randomly assigned to a diet. Weight gain was measured in grams after two weeks. Use an ANOVA to determine if the diets produce different results. If the ANOVA is significant, perform Scheffé tests on the individual comparisons.

Diet #1	Diet #2	Diet #3
18	26	16
13	19	13
12	30	11
19	23	11
15	27	16
16	23	15

2. To see if an exercise program developed for CV patients had any effect on pulse rate, an investigator measured the pulse rate of 10 patients before entering the program and after being in the program for 1, 4, and 12 weeks. Use an ANOVA to see if the program affected pulse rate.

Patient #	Start	1 week	4 weeks	12 weeks
1	90	87	88	90
2	80	80	78	74
3	70	75	73	75
4	76	82	75	72
5	82	80	74	70
6	85	83	80	76
7	100	95	85	82
8	80	82	75	75
9	90	95	82	80
10	75	75	70	72

Chapter 13
Chi Square

Parametric Versus
Nonparametric Statistics

The statistical tests discussed so far, z, t, F, and ANOVA, are **parametric tests.** In addition to requiring at least interval scale data, they all require, directly or indirectly, that certain assumptions be made about the underlying distributions before they may be used. In situations where $N < 30$, the t test and ANOVA require normal distributions and homogeneity of variances; where $N > 30$, the central limit theorem handles these problems for us.

Statistical tests that need only nominal or ordinal scale data are referred to as **nonparametric tests** or as **distribution-free statistics** since they require few, if any, assumptions about the underlying distributions. Generally nonparametric statistics are easier to compute and have wider application than parametric statistics. Often the statement is made that parametric statistics are more powerful than nonparametric statistics; this is true only if all the assumptions for the parametric statistic have been fulfilled. If we have unequal N's, lack homogeneity of variances, and have oppositely skewed distributions, the t test is usually not as powerful as converting the data to ordinal scale and using a nonparametric test.

Chi Square (χ^2)

We will begin our discussion of nonparametric tests with the chi square test (χ^2). Chi square is designed to be used when one has mutually exclusive and exhaustive categories and the data consists of frequency counts, that is, nominal scale data. Chi square is defined as the sum of the squared differences between the observed frequency and the expected frequency, divided by the expected frequency:

$$\chi^2 = \Sigma \frac{(O - E)^2}{E} \tag{13–1}$$

Expected Values Known

The state of Oregon is divided into three HSA's and Dr. M observed that during 1974 there were 1780 deaths from malignant neoplasms in area I, 1466 in area II, and 516 in area III (Table 13.1). In this instance we have frequency count data; we can not compute means and see if they differ across areas. Dr. M can use chi square to determine if the number of deaths from this cause differs significantly in the three areas. Of the total population in the state during 1974, 45% of the people resided in area I, 42% in area II, and 13% in area III. Therefore if the mortality rate from malignant neoplasms was the same in all areas, we would expect 45% of the deaths to have occurred in area I, 42% in area II, and 13% in area III.

Our computed value for chi square is 14.18 and is evaluated using Appendix D. To enter this table we need degrees of freedom which, in this case, are equal to the number of areas, minus one: $df = 3 - 1 = 2$. Entering Appendix D with $df = 2$ we find that the table value for alpha of .05 is 5.991. The decision rule for chi square is the same as that used for z, t, and ANOVA: if the computed value exceeds the table value for the chosen alpha level, we reject the null hypothesis. Here Dr. M would reject the null hypothesis and conclude that the areas do have significantly different mortality rates for malignant neoplasms.

In Chapter 10 we discussed several ways by which we could determine the probability of 8 female infants in 10 births. Chi square may also be used to test this hypothesis. We observed 8 girls and 2 boys; assuming a 50–50 split we would expect 5 girls and 5 boys so:

$$\chi^2 = \frac{(8 - 5)^2}{5} + \frac{(2 - 5)^2}{5} = 3.60$$

with $df = 2 - 1 = 1$.

Table 13.1.   *Chi square for malignant neoplasms*

Area	Observed	Expected	$O - E$	$(O - E)^2$	$(O - E)^2/E$
I	1780	$3762 \times .45 = 1693$	87	7,569	4.47
II	1466	$3762 \times .42 = 1580$	−114	12,996	8.22
III	516	$3762 \times .13 = 489$	27	729	1.49
					$14.18 = \chi^2$

However, as was the case when we used the z statistic with this data, we have discrete data and a continuous table. In cases where $df = 1$ and any of the expected values are less than 10, a correction for continuity should be applied to chi square. Typically Yate's correction, which consists of reducing the absolute values of the differences by 0.5, has been used:

$$\chi^2 = \Sigma \frac{(|O - E| - .5)^2}{E} \qquad (13\text{–}2)$$

so

$$\chi^2 = \frac{(|8 - 5| - .5)^2}{5} + \frac{(|2 - 5| - .5)^2}{5} = 2.50$$

It has been argued that Yate's correction is overly conservative, especially when applied to 2×2 tables. Given a 2×2 table with cell entries and row and column totals as shown in Table 13.2, the data may be analyzed by use of the formula:

$$\chi^2 = \frac{N(|AD - BC| - .5)^2}{JKLM} \qquad (13\text{–}3)$$

This formula does not necessitate the computation of expected values.

In situations where the expected values are two or less, chi square should not be used even with corrections. Fisher's exact method is preferred in this case (Siegel, 1956).

Table 13.2.   *General format for two by two table*

A	B	J
C	D	K
L	M	N

Contingency Tables

Thus far we have discussed the use of chi square in situations where we have had some basis for determining the expected values. Suppose that you want to determine if socioeconomic level influences whether parents have their children immunized for polio. You select an appropriate sample and classify people into three socioeconomic levels with the results shown in Table 13.3. Here you do not have a theory to predict what percentage of parents fall into each of your socioeconomic levels. You can generate the expected frequencies for each cell by calculating the product of the row and column totals of that cell and dividing this product by the total number of observations. In general, for a 2 × 3 data matrix the expected values are given in Table 13.4.

Calculating the expected values, we can compute χ^2 as shown in Table 13.5. The degrees of freedom for a chi square matrix 2 × 2 or larger are given by

$$df = (r - 1)(c - 1) \tag{13-4}$$

where:

r = the number of rows in the matrix

c = the number of columns in the matrix

In the present example $df = (2 - 1)(3 - 1) = 2$, and with $df = 2$, $\alpha = .05$, we find a value of 5.991 in Appendix D so that our chi square is significant. Hence there is a relationship between whether a child is immunized against polio and the socioeconomic level of his or her family. In the general case, a significant chi square tells us that there is a relationship between the row variable and the column variable; it does not tell us what kind of relationship exists. To determine this we must examine the differences between the observed and the expected frequencies. In our example we find that the biggest differences occur in the medium and low socioeconomic levels and that as socioeconomic level increases, the probability of immunization also increases.

Tests for Normality or Goodness of Fit

The chi square test may be used to determine if two distributions have the same shape or if a particular distribution deviates from normal. In the latter situation, the set of scores is normalized and the resulting distribution is used as the expected values against which the observed distribution is contrasted.

Table 13.3. *Effects of socioeconomic level upon frequency of polio immunizations*

| | Socioeconomic Level | | | |
	High	Medium	Low	
Immunized	160	500	300	960
Not Immunized	140	300	600	1040
	300	800	900	2000

Table 13.4. *Expected Chi Square values for contingency table*

AC/N	AD/N	AE/N	A
BC/N	BD/N	BE/N	B
C	D	E	N

Table 13.5. *Computation of Chi Square for socioeconomic data*

O	E	O − E	(O − E)²	(O − E)²/E
160	144	16	256	1.78
500	384	116	13,456	35.04
300	432	− 132	17,424	40.33
140	156	− 16	256	1.64
300	416	− 116	13,456	32.35
600	468	132	17,424	37.23
				148.37 = χ^2

Exercise 13

1. Eighty-eight patients were asked whether they were diabetics and 9 responded positively. Of the 88, 50 had a history of chronic heart disease (CHD). Use chi square to determine if there is a relationship between CHD and diabetes.

2. Three hundred sixty-two married women were interviewed as to the type of birth control methods that they used. They were asked if they were satisfied with the method that they used the most frequently, and the resulting data are recorded below. Is there any relationship between the method used and whether it is deemed successful?

	Satisfied	Unsatisfied
Rhythm	18	74
Pill	57	12
Coil	42	6
Other	123	30

Chapter 14
Other Distribution-Free Statistics

In the preceding chapter, the topic of distribution-free statistics was introduced with a discussion of chi square. The chi square test is designed for situations where we have two or more independent groups, nominal scale data, but the chi square distribution is the basis for many other distribution-free statistics. We shall consider other distribution-free statistics in this chapter starting first with tests designed for two sets of scores and then take up tests designed for three or more sets of scores.

Two Groups

Nominal Scale Data

Chi Square. As has just been indicated, in situations where we have two independent groups, nominal scale data, the chi square test may be used. This statistic should only be used if each expected value is greater than or equal to two, otherwise Fisher's exact method should be applied (Siegel, 1956).

Table 14.1.   *Two by two table*
for significant changes

		After	
		−	+
Before	+	A	B
	−	C	D

McNemar's Test for Significant Changes.   If we have nominal scale data and repeated measurements on the same individuals, McNemar's test for significant changes may be used. The data are summarized in a table such as Table 14.1 where plus and minus are used to designate different responses. McNemar's test consists of using the number of individuals who change their response from one testing to the next (+ to −, A or − to +, D) and has a chi square distribution. Because the test has one degree of freedom, it is corrected for continuity.

$$\chi^2 = \frac{(|A - D| - .5)^2}{A + D} \tag{14-1}$$

The Home Economics Department at OSU initiated a program to persuade housewives in the state to purchase the cheaper cuts of meat, such as tongue, brains, and kidney. They developed a short lecture and movie on the nutritional value of these cuts and how they can be tastefully prepared. In order to evaluate the effectiveness of this presentation, they gave 100 housewives a questionnaire to measure their attitudes toward these cuts. The housewives then viewed the presentation and filled out the questionnaire again. The results are given in Table 14.2 and are evaluated using McNemar's test.

$$\chi^2 = \frac{(|10 - 30| - .5)^2}{10 + 30} = 9.51$$

With $df = 1$ this is significant to $\alpha = .01$, and inspection of the raw data indicates that the presentation was effective in changing attitudes from negative to positive.

Table 14.2. *Effectiveness of the presentation in changing attitudes*

		Attitude After the Show	
		Positive	Negative
Attitude Before Show	Positive	10	10
	Negative	30	50

Ordinal Scale Data

Medians Test.   Dr. M wanted to determine if patients about to undergo open heart surgery were more anxious than patients about to undergo chest surgery. Using a five-point clinical judgment scale to measure anxiety, he tested 12 open heart patients and 14 chest surgery patients with the results given in Table 14.3.

Dr. M has two independent groups, ordinal scale measurement, and wants to test the null hypothesis that the medians of the two groups are equal. This may be done using the medians test. The first step is to determine the median anxiety level of all 26 patients regardless of group. In this case, the median is 3.5 since 13 scores are larger than this value and 13 are smaller. Next we determine the number of patients in each group who are above this value and the number below it. These values are used as the observed frequencies in a chi square (Table 14.4). The expected values are obtained by dividing the number of patients in each group by two (by definition the median should divide a group in half).

$$\chi^2 = \frac{(|5 - 6| - .5)^2}{6} + \frac{(|7 - 6| - .5)^2}{6} + \frac{(|8 - 7| - .5)^2}{7}$$

$$+ \frac{(|6 - 7| - .5)^2}{7} = 0.15$$

With $df = 1$ the null hypothesis is accepted. If it should happen that some of the scores fall on the median, then these are evenly split between above the median and below the median.

Table 14.3. *Anxiety levels of patients undergoing open heart surgery and chest surgery*

	\multicolumn{5}{c}{Anxiety Level}				
	1	2	3	4	5	
Open Heart	2	1	2	4	3	12
Chest	1	3	4	4	2	14

Table 14.4. *Number of open heart patients and chest surgery patients scoring above and below the median anxiety level*

	$<Md$	$>Md$
Open Heart	5	7
Chest	8	6

Mann-Whitney U.   The Mann-Whitney U test is also designed for ordinal scale data with two independent groups. This test is more powerful than the medians test but requires special tables that are not always available.

A blanching test has been developed as a tool in diagnosing coarctation of the aorta. You have collected recovery time data (in minutes) using this test for normal patients and for patients having coarctation. You would like to know if the average recovery time differs for these groups, but the groups have unequal N's and the variances differ significantly so you do not want to use the t test. We can test the null hypothesis that the two groups are from the same population using the U statistic. The first step is to rank all the scores regardless of group and then determine the sum of the ranks for each group. Next we compute U_1 and U_2. For the data in Table 14.5 we have:

$$U_1 = N_1 N_2 + \frac{N_1(N_1 + 1)}{2} - \Sigma R_1 \tag{14-2}$$

$$U_1 = 7(10) + \frac{7(8)}{2} - 86 = 12$$

Table 14.5.   *Blanching time for normal and coarctation patients*

Time for Coarctation Patients	Time for Normal Patients	Rank for Coarctations	Rank for Normals
4.50	1.50	17	10
3.00	1.15	15	7.5
1.10	2.25	5.5	12
1.10	1.75	5.5	11
3.00	1.00	15	2.5
3.00	1.00	15	2.5
2.50	1.25	13	9
	1.00		2.5
	1.00		2.5
	1.15		7.5
		$86 = \Sigma R_1$	$67 = \Sigma R_2$

$$U_2 = N_1 N_2 + \frac{N_2(N_2 + 1)}{2} - \Sigma R_2 \qquad (14\text{--}3)$$

$$U_2 = 7(10) + \frac{10(11)}{2} - 67 = 58$$

We select the smaller of U_1 and U_2 and turn to Appendix E. This table is entered using N_1 and N_2. In our example with N's of 7 and 10, we see that the table value for a two-tailed test at $\alpha = .05$ is 14. Since we select the smaller of the two U's, the decision rule for this test is: if the computed value for U is less than the table value, we reject the null hypothesis. U_1 is less than 14, so we reject the null hypothesis in our example.

Appendix E is applicable only when one of our samples has 9 or more observations but less than 20. If one group has more than 20 observations, U has a normal distribution and may be evaluated using the z statistic:

$$z = \frac{U - N_1 N_2/2}{\sqrt{\dfrac{N_1 N_2(N_1 + N_2 + 1)}{12}}} \qquad (14\text{--}4)$$

If both groups have 8 or fewer observations, the procedure is to rank all the scores in order of increasing size and to determine U_1 and U_2. In this case U_1 is the number of times a score grom group # 1 is preceded by a score from group #2 and, likewise, U_2 is the number of times a score from group #2 is preceded by a score from group #1. Again we select the smaller of U_1 and U_2 and enter Appendix F with the appropriate N.

Suppose our coarctation study had consisted of only the following data:

Coarctation:	4.5,	3.0,	1.1		
Normal:	1.5,	1.0,	1.15,	2.25,	1.75

Ordering these scores and identifying them as N or C we have:

1.00	1.10	1.15	1.50	1.75	2.25	3.00	4.50
N	C	N	N	N	N	C	C

To compute U_1 we see that 1.10 is preceded by one score from the normal group, 3.00 is preceded by five scores from the normal group, and 4.50 is preceded by five scores from the normal group, so:

$$U_1 = 1 + 5 + 5 = 11$$

likewise

$$U_2 = 0 + 1 + 1 + 1 + 1 = 4$$

U_2 is the smaller, and since there are 5 in the normal group, we enter Appendix F with $U_2 = 4$, $N_2 = 5$ and find a table value of 0.196. This is the probability of a one-tailed test, so we multiply this value by 2 to obtain the two-tailed probability: $2(0.196) = 0.392$. Thus the probability that the two samples came from the same population is 0.392.

Sign Test.   Now let us consider statistical tests that may be used when we have ordinal scale data and repeated measurements on the same group of subjects or matched pairs of subjects. The nurses on a particular ward were asked to make a point of speaking to each patient, asking the patients how they felt, calling them by name, wishing them good morning, etc. To see if this had any effect on how the patients perceived the nursing service that they were provided, each patient was asked to rate the quality of nursing care on a ten point scale the day before the program was begun and then again two days later. The data for 15 patients are given in Table 14.6.

The first test that we will consider is the sign test. Each pair of observations is examined, and we note whether the second member of each pair is larger (+), smaller (−), or the same (0) as the first member. Tied pairs are thrown out, and the sign occurring the smaller number of times is used as X in the z statistic:

$$z = \frac{|X - N/2| - .5}{.5 \sqrt{N}} \qquad (14\text{--}5)$$

Table 14.6. *Rating of nursing care*

Score before Start of Program	Score after Program Begun	Direction of Change	D	Rank
7	10	+	3	8
8	8	0	0	
7	9	+	2	5
7	7	0	0	
6	7	+	2	5
9	9	0	0	
7	10	+	3	8
7	7	0	0	
7	6	−	−1	−2
8	9	+	1	2
2	6	+	4	10
9	8	−	−1	−2
8	8	0	0	
6	9	+	3	8
5	6	+	2	5

Returning to the data in Table 14.6, we see from column #3 that 8 pairs increased from the first to the second measurement; 2 decreased; and 5 remained unchanged. Substituting these values into formula 14.5 we have:

$$z = \frac{|2 - 5| - .5}{.5 \sqrt{10}} = 1.58$$

The null hypothesis that is tested by the sign test is that the number of pairs that showed an increase is equal to the number of pairs that showed a decrease. Since 1.58 does not exceed ±1.96, we must accept the null hypothesis and conclude that the perception of the quality of nursing care did not change.

In cases where $N < 10$, the data should be evaluated by use of the binomial theorem.

Wilcoxon Matched-Pairs Signed-Rank Test.   The sign test uses only the direction of change between each pair of scores. The Wilcoxon test utilizes both the direction and magnitude of change and hence is a more powerful statistic. The first step in computing this statistic is to determine the numerical difference between each pair of scores. Using the data in Table 14.6 again, we have these values in column #4. Next we rank the absolute value of these difference scores and then determine the sum of the ranks for pairs that showed an increase and the sum for pairs that showed a decrease (column #5). The smaller of these two sums is evaluated using Appendix G. The data in Table 14.6 have a sum of 51 for the positive scores and a sum of 4 for the negative pairs. Entering Appendix G with $N = 10$, we find that a value of 8 or less is significant for an alpha of .05, two-tailed test. Since 4 is less than 8, we reject the null hypothesis using this test. The null hypothesis tested by the Wilcoxon test is that the sum of the positive ranks is equal to the sum of the negative ranks.

Three or More Groups

Nominal Scale Data

Chi Square. If we have nominal scale data, three or more sets of independent data, the chi square test may be used.

Cochran's Q. In cases involving correlated data, nominal scale measurements, Cochran's Q test may be applied.

Dr. O presented three pediatric cases to a nursing epidemiology class and asked each of the ten students to decide if the patient had rubella or not. Dr. O wishes to determine if there is any difference in the accuracy of diagnosis between the three cases. A correct diagnosis is given a score of one, and an incorrect diagnosis a score of zero. The data are recorded in Table 14.7. The formula for Cochran's Q is:

$$Q = \frac{(k - 1)[k\Sigma T_j^2 - (\Sigma L_i)^2]}{k\Sigma L_i - \Sigma L_i^2} \tag{14-6}$$

where:

k = the number of columns

L_i = the sum of all observations on line i

T_j = the sum of column j

Analyzing Dr. O's data we have:

$$Q = \frac{(3 - 1)\,[3(8^2 + 4^2 + 7^2) - 19^2]}{3(19) - 39} = 2.89$$

Q has a chi square distribution with $df = k - 1$. The null hypothesis in this situation is that the probability of a correct response is the same for each case, in other words, the sum of each of the columns is the same. With $df = 2$, $\alpha = .05$, Appendix D provides a value of 5.991, so Dr. O accepts the null hypothesis of no difference.

Table 14.7. *Diagnosis of three pediatric cases*

Student	Case I	Case II	Case III	L	L^2
1	1	0	1	2	4
2	1	1	0	2	4
3	1	0	0	1	1
4	0	1	1	2	4
5	1	0	1	2	4
6	1	0	1	2	4
7	1	0	0	1	1
8	0	1	1	2	4
9	1	1	1	3	9
10	1	0	1	2	4
	8	4	7	19	39

Ordinal Scale Data

Medians Test.   The medians test, which we have already discussed in analyzing ordinal scale data for two groups, may also be used when we have three or more sets of independent ordinal scale data.

Kruskal-Wallis H Test.   Another test that is more efficient in this type of situation is the Kruskal-Wallis one-way analysis of variance or *H* test. This statistic tests whether three or more independent samples have been drawn from the same population.

Dr. P has measured the amount of fluid consumed by three groups of rats during a week. One group of rats was given a .05% alcohol solution to drink, one group a 5% solution, and one group a 12% solution. The week's consumption in cc's is given in Table 14.8. Inspection of the data suggests that the variances and distributions of the three groups may be different. Given the small sample sizes, Dr. P decides that he would prefer to use a nonparametric test and chooses the Kruskal-Wallis *H* test.

The first step is to combine all the scores from the three groups and rank them. Next, the ranks are separated back into the original groups, and the sum of the ranks for each group is computed. This has been done in columns # 4, 5, and 6 in Table 14.8.

The formula for the Kruskal-Wallis test is:

$$H = \frac{12}{N(N + 1)}\left(\Sigma\frac{\Sigma R_j^2}{n_j}\right) - 3(N + 1) \qquad (14\text{–}7)$$

Table 14.8. *Alcohol solutions consumed by three groups of rats*

| cc's Consumed | | | Ranks | | |
.05%	5%	10%	.05%	5%	10%
150	110	40	14	8.5	1.5
180	120	50	17	10.5	3
130	110	60	13	8.5	5
170	100	55	15	7	4
175	130	65	16	12	6
	120	40		10.5	1.5
			$\Sigma R = 75$	57	21

where:

n_j = the number of observations in group j

N = the total number of observations in the experiment

R_j = the sum of the ranks for group j

Thus for Dr. P's data we have:

$$H = \frac{12}{17(18)} \left(\frac{75^2}{5} + \frac{57^2}{6} + \frac{21^2}{6} \right) - 3(18) = 14.24$$

When the n in each group is 5 or more, H has a chi square distribution with $df = k - 1$, so Dr. P could conclude that his groups consumed different amounts of fluid. If any of the n's are less than 5, then the H statistic should be evaluated using the special tables in Appendix I.

Friedman Two-Way Analysis of Variance.   In cases where we have correlated observations, ordinal scale data, the Friedman two-way analysis of variance may be used to determine if these sets of observations have been drawn from the same population. Dr. P found that his three groups of animals consumed different amounts of fluid during the week. In order to see if consumption changed over time, Dr. P added a control group (0% alcohol) and recorded the median consumption per week for each group for four weeks. These data are recorded in Table 14.9.

The first step is to rank the scores of each group separately. Letting a rank of one indicate the least amount drunk in each group, we have the data shown in Table 14.10.

Table 14.9.   *Median weekly fluid consumption*

Group	Week I	II	III	IV
0%	180	178	182	179
.5%	170	176	178	178
5.0%	115	114	112	110
10.0%	52.5	50	51	51

Table 14.10.   *Ranks of weekly fluid consumption*

Group	Week I	II	III	IV
0%	3	1	4	2
.5%	1	2	3.5	3.5
5.0%	4	3	2	1
10.0%	4	1	2.5	2.5
	12	7	12	9

The formula for the Friedman statistic is:

$$\chi_r^2 = \frac{12}{kN(k+1)} (\Sigma R_j^2) - 3N(k+1) \tag{14-8}$$

where:

k = the number of columns

N = the number of rows

R_j = the sum of the ranks for column j

χ_r^2 is distributed like chi square with $df = k - 1$ when $k \geq 3$, $N \geq 10$, or $k \geq 4$, $N \geq 4$; otherwise χ_r^2 is evaluated using a special table found in Appendix J.

For our example, Dr. P has:

$$\chi_r^2 = \frac{12}{4(4)(5)} (12^2 + 7^2 + 12^2 + 9^2) - 3(4)(5) = 2.70$$

With $df = 4 - 1 = 3$, Dr. P must accept the null hypothesis that the amounts consumed did not differ over the four-week period.

In our example the rows consisted of repeated measurements on different groups of subjects. The Friedman test may also be used when the row entries are repeated measurements on individual subjects rather than on groups of subjects.

Exercise 14

1. A questionnaire was given to 12 in-patients to determine their satisfaction with the food service. The questionnaire consisted of 10 questions. The patient was asked to score each question on a five-point scale (0 very unsatisfactory to 4 very satisfactory). After completing the questionnaire the patients were told that a new food service manager had just been hired and that the results of the questionnaires would be made available to him. Three days later the same questionnaire was given to the same 12 patients to see if they had noticed any change in the service. The scores are given below.
   (a) Analyze the data using the sign test.
   (b) Analyze the data using the Wilcoxon test.

1st test	2nd test
19	26
25	32
21	16
16	19
6	12
14	15
24	22
12	18
12	16
24	26
21	27
20	24

2. A twenty-point rating scale was developed to measure psychological disorientation. This scale was given to 12 open heart patients and 10 chest surgery patients two days following surgery. Use the Mann-Whitney U to determine if there is any difference between the two patient categories on this test.

   Open Heart: 14, 18, 9, 12, 11, 14, 9, 15, 8, 16, 17, 19
   Chest Surgery: 7, 4, 10, 15, 7, 5, 16, 9, 6, 15

3. Using the data in Exercise 12, problem #1, perform a Kruskal-Wallis *H* test.

4. Using the data in Exercise 12, problem #2, perform a Friedman test.

Chapter 15

Choosing a Statistic

Now that we have discussed the computational procedures and uses of a variety of statistics, let me try to outline a simple procedure to use in the selection of the appropriate statistic for a given situation. The first thing always to consider is the scale of measurement that has been used to collect the data.

If you are selecting a descriptive statistic, then you may need to consider the shape of the distribution of your scores in addition to the scale of measurement. In computing a measure of central tendency on interval or ratio scale data, the mean will be the most appropriate average to use if the data are normally distributed; if the data are skewed, the median should be used; if they are peaked, the mode.

In deciding upon an inferential statistic, two approaches may be taken. First we can use Table 15.1. To enter this table we need to know: (1) the scale of measurement used, (2) the number of groups being compared, k, and (3) whether the sets of scores are independent or repeated measurements. With this information we enter one of the cells in Table 15.1 and find the tests

Table 15.1. *Descriptive and inferential statistics*

		Descriptive	
Scales of Measurement	*Averages*	*Variability*	*Correlation*
Nominal	mode		phi
Ordinal	median	range	rho
		Q	
Interval	mean	SD	r
		s	r_b
		$s_{\bar{x}}$	multiple
			partial
			eta

	Inferential			
	k = 2		*k ≥ 3*	
	Independent	*Repeated*	*Independent*	*Repeated*
Nominal	chi square	McNemar	chi square	Cochran's Q
Ordinal	median test	Sign test	median test	Friedman
	Mann-Whitney	Wilcoxon	Kruskal-Wallis H	
Interval	z	z	ANOVA	ANOVA
	t test	t test	Scheffé	Scheffé
	F			

that may be used. Remember, however, that some of these tests have assumptions associated with them and it may be necessary to rescale your data and move vertically within a column. For instance, if you have two sets of 15 independent observations each, interval scale data, but the two distributions are oppositely skewed and lack homogeneity of variance, you can not use a t test. However, you can rank these scores and thus convert them to ordinal scale data and use a Mann-Whitney U test which does not require normal distributions or homogeneity of variance.

A second approach is to consider the null hypothesis that you wish to test. Table 15.2 lists the various inferential statistics covered in this text and the hypotheses that they may be used to test. Again note that some of these statistics have underlying assumptions that must be satisfied.

Table 15.2.   *Null hypotheses and inferential statistics*

Statistic	Null Hypotheses	
z	$X = \mu$	
	$\overline{X} = \mu$	
	$\mu_1 = \mu_2$	Independent or repeated, $N \geq 30$
	$r = 0$	$N \geq 30$
	$r_1 = r_2$	Independent
t test	$\mu_1 = \mu_2$	Independent or repeated, $N < 30$
	$r = 0$	$N < 30$
	$r_1 = r_2$	Correlated
	$b_y = 0$	
	$b_{y_1} = b_{y_2}$	
	$\rho = 0$	
	$r_{pb} = 0$	
	$r_b = 0$	
F	$\sigma_1^2 = \sigma_2^2$	
	$\eta = 0$	
ANOVA	$\mu_1 = \mu_2 = \mu_3 \cdots = \mu_k$	
Scheffé	$\mu_1 = \mu_2$	
Median test	$Md_1 = Md_2 = \cdots = Md_k$	
Mann-Whitney U	Two independent groups are from the same population	
Sign test	Number of pairs showing an increase equal the number showing a decrease	
Wilcoxon	Two matched sets of scores are from the same population	
Kruskal-Wallis	k samples are from the same population	
Friedman	k samples are from the same population	
Chi square	No difference exists between k-independent groups. phi $= 0$	
McNemar	Number of scores showing a positive change equals the number of scores showing a negative change	
Cochran's Q	k-matched sets of frequencies are not different	

Appendixes

Appendix A

Areas and ordinates of the normal curve

z	Area from μ to z	Area in Larger Portion	Area in Smaller Portion	Ordinate at z
0.00	.0000	.5000	.5000	.3989
0.01	.0040	.5040	.4960	.3989
0.02	.0080	.5080	.4920	.3989
0.03	.0120	.5120	.4880	.3988
0.04	.0160	.5160	.4840	.3986
0.05	.0199	.5199	.4801	.3984
0.06	.0239	.5239	.4761	.3982
0.07	.0279	.5279	.4721	.3980
0.08	.0319	.5319	.4681	.3977
0.09	.0359	.5359	.4641	.3973
0.10	.0398	.5398	.4602	.3970
0.11	.0438	.5438	.4562	.3965
0.12	.0478	.5478	.4522	.3961
0.13	.0517	.5517	.4483	.3956
0.14	.0557	.5557	.4443	.3951
0.15	.0596	.5596	.4404	.3945
0.16	.0636	.5636	.4364	.3939
0.17	.0675	.5675	.4325	.3932
0.18	.0714	.5714	.4286	.3925
0.19	.0753	.5753	.4247	.3918
0.20	.0793	.5793	.4207	.3910
0.21	.0832	.5832	.4168	.3902
0.22	.0871	.5871	.4129	.3894
0.23	.0910	.5910	.4090	.3885
0.24	.0948	.5948	.4052	.3876
0.25	.0987	.5987	.4013	.3867
0.26	.1026	.6026	.3974	.3857
0.27	.1064	.6064	.3936	.3847
0.28	.1103	.6103	.3897	.3836
0.29	.1141	.6141	.3859	.3825
0.30	.1179	.6179	.3821	.3814
0.31	.1217	.6217	.3783	.3802
0.32	.1255	.6255	.3745	.3790
0.33	.1293	.6293	.3707	.3778
0.34	.1331	.6331	.3669	.3765

Source: From Table 1 of E. S. Pearson and H. O. Hartley: *Biometrika Tables for Statisticians*, 3rd ed., vol. 1 (Cambridge: Cambridge University Press, 1970), by permission of the Biometrika Trustees.

Areas and ordinates of the normal curve (continued)

z	Area from μ to z	Area in Larger Portion	Area in Smaller Portion	Ordinate at z
0.35	.1368	.6368	.3632	.3752
0.36	.1406	.6406	.3594	.3739
0.37	.1443	.6443	.3557	.3725
0.38	.1480	.6480	.3520	.3712
0.39	.1517	.6517	.3483	.3697
0.40	.1554	.6554	.3446	.3683
0.41	.1591	.6591	.3409	.3668
0.42	.1628	.6628	.3372	.3653
0.43	.1664	.6664	.3336	.3637
0.44	.1700	.6700	.3300	.3621
0.45	.1736	.6736	.3264	.3605
0.46	.1772	.6772	.3228	.3589
0.47	.1808	.6808	.3192	.3572
0.48	.1844	.6844	.3156	.3555
0.49	.1879	.6879	.3121	.3538
0.50	.1915	.6915	.3085	.3521
0.51	.1950	.6950	.3050	.3503
0.52	.1985	.6985	.3015	.3485
0.53	.2019	.7019	.2981	.3467
0.54	.2054	.7054	.2946	.3448
0.55	.2088	.7088	.2912	.3429
0.56	.2123	.7123	.2877	.3410
0.57	.2157	.7157	.2843	.3391
0.58	.2190	.7190	.2810	.3372
0.59	.2224	.7224	.2776	.3352
0.60	.2257	.7257	.2743	.3332
0.61	.2291	.7291	.2709	.3312
0.62	.2324	.7324	.2676	.3292
0.63	.2357	.7357	.2643	.3271
0.64	.2389	.7389	.2611	.3251
0.65	.2422	.7422	.2578	.3230
0.66	.2454	.7454	.2546	.3209
0.67	.2486	.7486	.2514	.3187
0.68	.2517	.7517	.2483	.3166
0.69	.2549	.7549	.2451	.3144
0.70	.2580	.7580	.2420	.3123
0.71	.2611	.7611	.2389	.3101
0.72	.2642	.7642	.2358	.3079
0.73	.2673	.7673	.2327	.3056

Areas and ordinates of the normal curve (continued)

z	Area from μ to z	Area in Larger Portion	Area in Smaller Portion	Ordinate at z
0.74	.2704	.7704	.2296	.3034
0.75	.2734	.7734	.2266	.3011
0.76	.2764	.7764	.2236	.2989
0.77	.2794	.7794	.2206	.2966
0.78	.2823	.7823	.2177	.2943
0.79	.2852	.7852	.2148	.2920
0.80	.2881	.7881	.2119	.2897
0.81	.2910	.7910	.2090	.2874
0.82	.2939	.7939	.2061	.2850
0.83	.2967	.7967	.2033	.2827
0.84	.2995	.7995	.2005	.2803
0.85	.3023	.8023	.1977	.2780
0.86	.3051	.8051	.1949	.2756
0.87	.3078	.8078	.1922	.2732
0.88	.3106	.8106	.1894	.2709
0.89	.3133	.8133	.1867	.2685
0.90	.3159	.8159	.1841	.2661
0.91	.3186	.8186	.1814	.2637
0.92	.3212	.8212	.1788	.2613
0.93	.3238	.8238	.1762	.2589
0.94	.3264	.8264	.1736	.2565
0.95	.3289	.8289	.1711	.2541
0.96	.3315	.8315	.1685	.2516
0.97	.3340	.8340	.1660	.2492
0.98	.3365	.8365	.1635	.2468
0.99	.3389	.8389	.1611	.2444
1.00	.3413	.8413	.1587	.2420
1.01	.3438	.8438	.1562	.2396
1.02	.3461	.8461	.1539	.2371
1.03	.3485	.8485	.1515	.2347
1.04	.3508	.8508	.1492	.2323
1.05	.3531	.8531	.1469	.2299
1.06	.3554	.8554	.1446	.2275
1.07	.3577	.8577	.1423	.2251
1.08	.3599	.8599	.1401	.2227
1.09	.3621	.8621	.1379	.2203
1.10	.3643	.8643	.1357	.2179
1.11	.3665	.8665	.1335	.2155
1.12	.3686	.8686	.1314	.2131

Areas and ordinates of the normal curve (continued)

z	Area from μ to z	Area in Larger Portion	Area in Smaller Portion	Ordinate at z
1.13	.3708	.8708	.1292	.2107
1.14	.3729	.8729	.1271	.2083
1.15	.3749	.8749	.1251	.2059
1.16	.3770	.8770	.1230	.2036
1.17	.3790	.8790	.1210	.2012
1.18	.3810	.8810	.1190	.1989
1.19	.3830	.8830	.1170	.1965
1.20	.3849	.8849	.1151	.1942
1.21	.3869	.8869	.1131	.1919
1.22	.3888	.8888	.1112	.1895
1.23	.3907	.8907	.1093	.1872
1.24	.3925	.8925	.1075	.1849
1.25	.3944	.8944	.1056	.1826
1.26	.3962	.8962	.1038	.1804
1.27	.3980	.8980	.1020	.1781
1.28	.3997	.8997	.1003	.1758
1.29	.4015	.9015	.0985	.1736
1.30	.4032	.9032	.0968	.1714
1.31	.4049	.9049	.0951	.1691
1.32	.4066	.9066	.0934	.1669
1.33	.4082	.9082	.0918	.1647
1.34	.4099	.9099	.0901	.1626
1.35	.4115	.9115	.0885	.1604
1.36	.4131	.9131	.0869	.1582
1.37	.4147	.9147	.0853	.1561
1.38	.4162	.9162	.0838	.1539
1.39	.4177	.9177	.0823	.1518
1.40	.4192	.9192	.0808	.1497
1.41	.4207	.9207	.0793	.1476
1.42	.4222	.9222	.0778	.1456
1.43	.4236	.9236	.0764	.1435
1.44	.4251	.9251	.0749	.1415
1.45	.4265	.9265	.0735	.1394
1.46	.4279	.9279	.0721	.1374
1.47	.4292	.9292	.0708	.1354
1.48	.4306	.9306	.0694	.1334
1.49	.4319	.9319	.0681	.1315
1.50	.4332	.9332	.0668	.1295

Areas and ordinates of the normal curve (continued)

z	Area from μ to z	Area in Larger Portion	Area in Smaller Portion	Ordinate at z
1.51	.4345	.9345	.0655	.1276
1.52	.4357	.9357	.0643	.1257
1.53	.4370	.9370	.0630	.1238
1.54	.4382	.9382	.0618	.1219
1.55	.4394	.9394	.0606	.1200
1.56	.4406	.9406	.0594	.1182
1.57	.4418	.9418	.0582	.1163
1.58	.4429	.9429	.0571	.1145
1.59	.4441	.9441	.0559	.1127
1.60	.4452	.9452	.0548	.1109
1.61	.4463	.9463	.0537	.1092
1.62	.4474	.9474	.0526	.1074
1.63	.4484	.9484	.0516	.1057
1.64	.4495	.9495	.0505	.1040
1.65	.4505	.9505	.0495	.1023
1.66	.4515	.9515	.0485	.1006
1.67	.4525	.9525	.0475	.0989
1.68	.4535	.9535	.0465	.0973
1.69	.4545	.9545	.0455	.0957
1.70	.4554	.9554	.0446	.0940
1.71	.4564	.9564	.0436	.0925
1.72	.4573	.9573	.0427	.0909
1.73	.4582	.9582	.0418	.0893
1.74	.4591	.9591	.0409	.0878
1.75	.4599	.9599	.0401	.0863
1.76	.4608	.9608	.0392	.0848
1.77	.4616	.9616	.0384	.0833
1.78	.4625	.9625	.0375	.0818
1.79	.4633	.9633	.0367	.0804
1.80	.4641	.9641	.0359	.0790
1.81	.4649	.9649	.0351	.0775
1.82	.4656	.9656	.0344	.0761
1.83	.4664	.9664	.0336	.0748
1.84	.4671	.9671	.0329	.0734
1.85	.4678	.9678	.0322	.0721
1.86	.4686	.9686	.0314	.0707
1.87	.4693	.9693	.0307	.0694
1.88	.4699	.9699	.0301	.0681

Areas and ordinates of the normal curve (continued)

z	Area from μ to z	Area in Larger Portion	Area in Smaller Portion	Ordinate at z
1.89	.4706	.9706	.0294	.0669
1.90	.4713	.9713	.0287	.0656
1.91	.4719	.9719	.0281	.0644
1.92	.4726	.9726	.0274	.0632
1.93	.4732	.9732	.0268	.0620
1.94	.4738	.9738	.0262	.0608
1.95	.4744	.9744	.0256	.0596
1.96	.4750	.9750	.0250	.0584
1.97	.4756	.9756	.0244	.0573
1.98	.4761	.9761	.0239	.0562
1.99	.4767	.9767	.0233	.0551
2.00	.4772	.9772	.0228	.0540
2.01	.4778	.9778	.0222	.0529
2.02	.4783	.9783	.0217	.0519
2.03	.4788	.9788	.0212	.0508
2.04	.4793	.9793	.0207	.0498
2.05	.4798	.9798	.0202	.0488
2.06	.4803	.9803	.0197	.0478
2.07	.4808	.9808	.0192	.0468
2.08	.4812	.9812	.0188	.0459
2.09	.4817	.9817	.0183	.0449
2.10	.4821	.9821	.0179	.0440
2.11	.4826	.9826	.0174	.0431
2.12	.4830	.9830	.0170	.0422
2.13	.4834	.9834	.0166	.0413
2.14	.4838	.9838	.0162	.0404
2.15	.4842	.9842	.0158	.0396
2.16	.4846	.9846	.0154	.0387
2.17	.4850	.9850	.0150	.0379
2.18	.4854	.9854	.0146	.0371
2.19	.4857	.9857	.0143	.0363
2.20	.4861	.9861	.0139	.0355
2.21	.4864	.9864	.0136	.0347
2.22	.4868	.9868	.0132	.0339
2.23	.4871	.9871	.0129	.0332
2.24	.4875	.9875	.0125	.0325
2.25	.4878	.9878	.0122	.0317
2.26	.4881	.9881	.0119	.0310
2.27	.4884	.9884	.0116	.0303

Areas and ordinates of the normal curve (continued)

z	Area from μ to z	Area in Larger Portion	Area in Smaller Portion	Ordinate at z
2.28	.4887	.9887	.0113	.0297
2.29	.4890	.9890	.0110	.0290
2.30	.4893	.9893	.0107	.0283
2.31	.4896	.9896	.0104	.0277
2.32	.4898	.9898	.0102	.0270
2.33	.4901	.9901	.0099	.0264
2.34	.4904	.9904	.0096	.0258
2.35	.4906	.9906	.0094	.0252
2.36	.4909	.9909	.0091	.0246
2.37	.4911	.9911	.0089	.0241
2.38	.4913	.9913	.0087	.0235
2.39	.4916	.9916	.0084	.0229
2.40	.4918	.9918	.0082	.0224
2.41	.4920	.9920	.0080	.0219
2.42	.4922	.9922	.0078	.0213
2.43	.4925	.9925	.0075	.0208
2.44	.4927	.9927	.0073	.0203
2.45	.4929	.9929	.0071	.0198
2.46	.4931	.9931	.0069	.0194
2.47	.4932	.9932	.0068	.0189
2.48	.4934	.9934	.0066	.0184
2.49	.4936	.9936	.0064	.0180
2.50	.4938	.9938	.0062	.0175
2.51	.4940	.9940	.0060	.0171
2.52	.4941	.9941	.0059	.0167
2.53	.4943	.9943	.0057	.0163
2.54	.4945	.9945	.0055	.0158
2.55	.4946	.9946	.0054	.0154
2.56	.4948	.9948	.0052	.0151
2.57	.4949	.9949	.0051	.0147
2.58	.4951	.9951	.0049	.0143
2.59	.4952	.9952	.0048	.0139
2.60	.4953	.9953	.0047	.0136
2.61	.4955	.9955	.0045	.0132
2.62	.4956	.9956	.0044	.0129
2.63	.4957	.9957	.0043	.0126
2.64	.4959	.9959	.0041	.0122
2.65	.4960	.9960	.0040	.0119
2.66	.4961	.9961	.0039	.0116

*Areas and ordinates of the normal curve (*continued*)*

z	Area from μ to z	Area in Larger Portion	Area in Smaller Portion	Ordinate at z
2.67	.4962	.9962	.0038	.0113
2.68	.4963	.9963	.0037	.0110
2.69	.4964	.9964	.0036	.0107
2.70	.4965	.9965	.0035	.0104
2.71	.4966	.9966	.0034	.0101
2.72	.4967	.9967	.0033	.0099
2.73	.4968	.9968	.0032	.0096
2.74	.4969	.9969	.0031	.0093
2.75	.4970	.9970	.0030	.0091
2.76	.4971	.9971	.0029	.0088
2.77	.4972	.9972	.0028	.0086
2.78	.4973	.9973	.0027	.0084
2.79	.4974	.9974	.0026	.0081
2.80	.4974	.9974	.0026	.0079
2.81	.4975	.9975	.0025	.0077
2.82	.4976	.9976	.0024	.0075
2.83	.4977	.9977	.0023	.0073
2.84	.4977	.9977	.0023	.0071
2.85	.4978	.9978	.0022	.0069
2.86	.4979	.9979	.0021	.0067
2.87	.4979	.9979	.0021	.0065
2.88	.4980	.9980	.0020	.0063
2.89	.4981	.9981	.0019	.0061
2.90	.4981	.9981	.0019	.0060
2.91	.4982	.9982	.0018	.0058
2.92	.4982	.9982	.0018	.0056
2.93	.4983	.9983	.0017	.0055
2.94	.4984	.9984	.0016	.0053
2.95	.4984	.9984	.0016	.0051
2.96	.4985	.9985	.0015	.0050
2.97	.4985	.9985	.0015	.0048
2.98	.4986	.9986	.0014	.0047
2.99	.4986	.9986	.0014	.0046
3.00	.4987	.9987	.0013	.0044
3.01	.4987	.9987	.0013	.0043
3.02	.4987	.9987	.0013	.0042
3.03	.4988	.9988	.0012	.0040
3.04	.4988	.9988	.0012	.0039

Areas and ordinates of the normal curve (continued)

z	Area from μ to z	Area in Larger Portion	Area in Smaller Portion	Ordinate at z
3.05	.4989	.9989	.0011	.0038
3.06	.4989	.9989	.0011	.0037
3.07	.4989	.9989	.0011	.0036
3.08	.4990	.9990	.0010	.0035
3.09	.4990	.9990	.0010	.0034
3.10	.4990	.9990	.0010	.0033
3.11	.4991	.9991	.0009	.0032
3.12	.4991	.9991	.0009	.0031
3.13	.4991	.9991	.0009	.0030
3.14	.4992	.9992	.0008	.0029
3.15	.4992	.9992	.0008	.0028
3.16	.4992	.9992	.0008	.0027
3.17	.4992	.9992	.0008	.0026
3.18	.4993	.9993	.0007	.0025
3.19	.4993	.9993	.0007	.0025
3.20	.4993	.9993	.0007	.0024
3.21	.4993	.9993	.0007	.0023
3.22	.4994	.9994	.0006	.0022
3.23	.4994	.9994	.0006	.0022
3.24	.4994	.9994	.0006	.0021
3.30	.4995	.9995	.0005	.0017
3.40	.4997	.9997	.0003	.0012
3.50	.4998	.9998	.0002	.0009
3.60	.4998	.9998	.0002	.0006
3.70	.4999	.9999	.0001	.0004
3.80	.4999277	.9999277	.0000723	.000292
3.90	.4999519	.9999519	.0000481	.000199
4.00	.4999683	.9999683	.0000317	.000134
4.10	.4999793	.9999793	.0000207	.000089
4.20	.4999867	.9999867	.0000133	.000059
4.30	.4999915	.9999915	.0000085	.000039
4.40	.4999946	.9999946	.0000054	.000025
4.50	.4999966	.9999966	.0000034	.000016
4.60	.4999979	.9999979	.0000021	.000010
4.70	.4999987	.9999987	.0000013	.000006
4.80	.4999992	.9999992	.0000008	.000004
4.90	.4999995	.9999995	.0000005	.000002
5.00	.4999997	.9999997	.0000003	.000001

Appendix B

Distribution of t

df	.9	.8	.7	.6	.5	.4	.3	.2	.1	.05	.02	.01	.001
							Probability						
1	.158	.325	.510	.727	1.000	1.376	1.963	3.078	6.314	12.706	31.821	63.657	636.619
2	.142	.289	.445	.617	.816	1.061	1.386	1.886	2.920	4.303	6.965	9.925	31.598
3	.137	.277	.424	.584	.765	.978	1.250	1.638	2.353	3.182	4.541	5.841	12.924
4	.134	.271	.414	.569	.741	.941	1.190	1.533	2.132	2.776	3.747	4.604	8.610
5	.132	.267	.408	.559	.727	.920	1.156	1.476	2.015	2.571	3.365	4.032	6.869
6	.131	.265	.404	.553	.718	.906	1.134	1.440	1.943	2.447	3.143	3.707	5.959
7	.130	.263	.402	.549	.711	.896	1.119	1.415	1.895	2.365	2.998	3.499	5.408
8	.130	.262	.399	.546	.706	.889	1.108	1.397	1.860	2.306	2.896	3.355	5.041
9	.129	.261	.398	.543	.703	.883	1.100	1.383	1.833	2.262	2.821	3.250	4.781
10	.129	.260	.397	.542	.700	.879	1.093	1.372	1.812	2.228	2.764	3.169	4.587
11	.129	.260	.396	.540	.697	.876	1.088	1.363	1.796	2.201	2.718	3.106	4.437
12	.128	.259	.395	.539	.695	.873	1.083	1.356	1.782	2.179	2.681	3.055	4.318
13	.128	.259	.394	.538	.694	.870	1.079	1.350	1.771	2.160	2.650	3.012	4.221
14	.128	.258	.393	.537	.692	.868	1.076	1.345	1.761	2.145	2.624	2.977	4.140
15	.128	.258	.393	.536	.691	.866	1.074	1.341	1.753	2.131	2.602	2.947	4.073
16	.128	.258	.392	.535	.690	.865	1.071	1.337	1.746	2.120	2.583	2.921	4.015
17	.128	.257	.392	.534	.689	.863	1.069	1.333	1.740	2.110	2.567	2.898	3.965
18	.127	.257	.392	.534	.688	.862	1.067	1.330	1.734	2.101	2.552	2.878	3.922
19	.127	.257	.391	.533	.688	.861	1.066	1.328	1.729	2.093	2.539	2.861	3.883
20	.127	.257	.391	.533	.687	.860	1.064	1.325	1.725	2.086	2.528	2.845	3.850
21	.127	.257	.391	.532	.686	.859	1.063	1.323	1.721	2.080	2.518	2.831	3.819
22	.127	.256	.390	.532	.686	.858	1.061	1.321	1.717	2.074	2.508	2.819	3.792
23	.127	.256	.390	.532	.685	.858	1.060	1.319	1.714	2.069	2.500	2.807	3.767
24	.127	.256	.390	.531	.685	.857	1.059	1.318	1.711	2.064	2.492	2.797	3.745
25	.127	.256	.390	.531	.684	.856	1.058	1.316	1.708	2.060	2.485	2.787	3.725
26	.127	.256	.390	.531	.684	.856	1.058	1.315	1.706	2.056	2.479	2.779	3.707
27	.127	.256	.389	.531	.684	.855	1.057	1.314	1.703	2.052	2.473	2.771	3.690
28	.127	.256	.389	.530	.683	.855	1.056	1.313	1.701	2.048	2.467	2.763	3.674
29	.127	.256	.389	.530	.683	.854	1.055	1.311	1.699	2.045	2.462	2.756	3.659
30	.127	.256	.389	.530	.683	.854	1.055	1.310	1.697	2.042	2.457	2.750	3.646
40	.126	.255	.388	.529	.681	.851	1.050	1.303	1.684	2.021	2.423	2.704	3.551
60	.126	.254	.387	.527	.679	.848	1.046	1.296	1.671	2.000	2.390	2.660	3.460
120	.126	.254	.386	.526	.677	.845	1.041	1.289	1.658	1.980	2.358	2.617	3.373
∝	.126	.253	.385	.524	.674	.842	1.036	1.282	1.645	1.960	2.326	2.576	3.291

Source: From Table III of R. A. Fisher and F. Yates, *Statistical Tables for Biological, Agricultural and Medical Research*, 6th ed. (London: Longman Group Ltd., 1970), (previously published by Oliver and Boyd, Edinburgh), by permission of the authors and publishers.

Appendix C

Distribution of F

| df denom. | α | \multicolumn{7}{c}{df *for Numerator*} |
		1	2	3	4	5	6	7
1	.10	39.86	49.50	53.59	55.83	57.24	58.20	58.91
	.05	161.40	199.50	215.70	224.60	230.20	234.00	236.80
	.01	4052.00	4999.50	5403.00	5625.00	5764.00	5859.00	5928.00
2	.10	8.53	9.00	9.16	9.24	9.29	9.33	9.35
	.05	18.51	19.00	19.16	19.25	19.30	19.33	19.35
	.01	98.50	99.00	99.17	99.25	99.30	99.33	99.36
3	.10	5.54	5.46	5.39	5.34	5.31	5.28	5.27
	.05	10.13	9.55	9.28	9.12	9.01	8.94	8.89
	.01	34.12	30.82	29.46	28.71	28.24	27.91	27.67
4	.10	4.54	4.32	4.19	4.11	4.05	4.01	3.98
	.05	7.71	6.94	6.59	6.39	6.26	6.16	6.09
	.01	21.20	18.00	16.69	15.98	15.52	15.21	14.98
5	.10	4.06	3.78	3.62	3.52	3.45	3.40	3.37
	.05	6.61	5.79	5.41	5.19	5.05	4.95	4.88
	.01	16.26	13.27	12.06	11.39	10.97	10.67	10.46
6	.10	3.78	3.46	3.29	3.18	3.11	3.05	3.01
	.05	5.99	5.14	4.76	4.53	4.39	4.28	4.21
	.01	13.75	10.92	9.78	9.15	8.75	8.47	8.26
7	.10	3.59	3.26	3.07	2.96	2.88	2.83	2.78
	.05	5.59	4.74	4.35	4.12	3.97	3.87	3.79
	.01	12.25	9.55	8.45	7.85	7.46	7.19	6.99
8	.10	3.46	3.11	2.92	2.81	2.73	2.67	2.62
	.05	5.32	4.46	4.07	3.84	3.69	3.58	3.50
	.01	11.26	8.65	7.59	7.01	6.63	6.37	6.18
9	.10	3.36	3.01	2.81	2.69	2.61	2.55	2.51
	.05	5.12	4.26	3.86	3.63	3.48	3.37	3.29
	.01	10.56	8.02	6.99	6.42	6.06	5.80	5.61

Source: Abridged from Table 18 of E. S. Pearson and H. O. Hartley, *Biometrika Tables for Statisticians*, 3rd ed., vol. 1 (Cambridge: Cambridge University Press, 1970), by permission of the Biometrika Trustees.

Distribution of F *(continued)*

df denom.	α	1	2	3	4	5	6	7
10	.10	3.29	2.92	2.73	2.61	2.52	2.46	2.41
	.05	4.96	4.10	3.71	3.48	3.33	3.22	3.14
	.01	10.04	7.56	6.55	5.99	5.64	5.39	5.20
11	.10	3.23	2.86	2.66	2.54	2.45	2.39	2.34
	.05	4.84	3.98	3.59	3.36	3.20	3.09	3.01
	.01	9.65	7.21	6.22	5.67	5.32	5.07	4.89
12	.10	3.18	2.81	2.61	2.48	2.39	2.33	2.28
	.05	4.75	3.89	3.49	3.26	3.11	3.00	2.91
	.01	9.33	6.93	5.95	5.41	5.06	4.82	4.64
13	.10	3.14	2.76	2.56	2.43	2.35	2.28	2.23
	.05	4.67	3.81	3.41	3.18	3.03	2.92	2.83
	.01	9.07	6.70	5.74	5.21	4.86	4.62	4.44
14	.10	3.10	2.73	2.52	2.39	2.31	2.24	2.19
	.05	4.60	3.74	3.34	3.11	2.96	2.85	2.76
	.01	8.86	6.51	5.56	5.04	4.69	4.46	4.28
15	.10	3.07	2.70	2.49	2.36	2.27	2.21	2.16
	.05	4.54	3.68	3.29	3.06	2.90	2.79	2.71
	.01	8.68	6.36	5.42	4.89	4.56	4.32	4.14
16	.10	3.05	2.67	2.46	2.33	2.24	2.18	2.13
	.05	4.49	3.63	3.24	3.01	2.85	2.74	2.66
	.01	8.53	6.23	5.29	4.77	4.44	4.20	4.03
17	.10	3.03	2.64	2.44	2.31	2.22	2.15	2.10
	.05	4.45	3.59	3.20	2.96	2.81	2.70	2.61
	.01	8.40	6.11	5.18	4.67	4.34	4.10	3.93
18	.10	3.01	2.62	2.42	2.29	2.20	2.13	2.08
	.05	4.41	3.55	3.16	2.93	2.77	2.66	2.58
	.01	8.29	6.01	5.09	4.58	4.25	4.01	3.84

df *for Numerator*

Distribution of F *(continued)*

| df denom. | α | \multicolumn{7}{c}{df *for Numerator*} |
		1	2	3	4	5	6	7
19	.10	2.99	2.61	2.40	2.27	2.18	2.11	2.06
	.05	4.38	3.52	3.13	2.90	2.74	2.63	2.54
	.01	8.18	5.93	5.01	4.50	4.17	3.94	3.77
20	.10	2.97	2.59	2.38	2.25	2.16	2.09	2.04
	.05	4.35	3.49	3.10	2.87	2.71	2.60	2.51
	.01	8.10	5.85	4.94	4.43	4.10	3.87	3.70
21	.10	2.96	2.57	2.36	2.23	2.14	2.08	2.02
	.05	4.32	3.47	3.07	2.84	2.68	2.57	2.49
	.01	8.02	5.78	4.87	4.37	4.04	3.81	3.64
22	.10	2.95	2.56	2.35	2.22	2.13	2.06	2.01
	.05	4.30	3.44	3.05	2.82	2.66	2.55	2.46
	.01	7.95	5.72	4.82	4.31	3.99	3.76	3.59
23	.10	2.94	2.55	2.34	2.21	2.11	2.05	1.99
	.05	4.28	3.42	3.03	2.80	2.64	2.53	2.44
	.01	7.88	5.66	4.76	4.26	3.94	3.71	3.54
24	.10	2.93	2.54	2.33	2.19	2.10	2.04	1.98
	.05	4.26	3.40	3.01	2.78	2.62	2.51	2.42
	.01	7.82	5.61	4.72	4.22	3.90	3.67	3.50
25	.10	2.92	2.53	2.32	2.18	2.09	2.02	1.97
	.05	4.24	3.39	2.99	2.76	2.60	2.49	2.40
	.01	7.77	5.57	4.68	4.18	3.85	3.63	3.46
26	.10	2.91	2.52	2.31	2.17	2.08	2.01	1.96
	.05	4.23	3.37	2.98	2.74	2.59	2.47	2.39
	.01	7.72	5.53	4.64	4.14	3.82	3.59	3.42
27	.10	2.90	2.51	2.30	2.17	2.07	2.00	1.95
	.05	4.21	3.35	2.96	2.73	2.57	2.46	2.37
	.01	7.68	5.49	4.60	4.11	3.78	3.56	3.39

Distribution of F *(continued)*

df denom.	α	df *for Numerator*						
		1	2	3	4	5	6	7
28	.10	2.89	2.50	2.29	2.16	2.06	2.00	1.94
	.05	4.20	3.34	2.95	2.71	2.56	2.45	2.36
	.01	7.64	5.45	4.57	4.07	3.75	3.53	3.36
29	.10	2.89	2.50	2.28	2.15	2.06	1.99	1.93
	.05	4.18	3.33	2.93	2.70	2.55	2.43	2.35
	.01	7.60	5.42	4.54	4.04	3.73	3.50	3.33
30	.10	2.88	2.49	2.28	2.14	2.05	1.98	1.93
	.05	4.17	3.32	2.92	2.69	2.53	2.42	2.33
	.01	7.56	5.39	4.51	4.02	3.70	3.47	3.30
40	.10	2.84	2.44	2.23	2.09	2.00	1.93	1.87
	.05	4.08	3.23	2.84	2.61	2.45	2.34	2.25
	.01	7.31	5.18	4.31	3.83	3.51	3.29	3.12
60	.10	2.79	2.39	2.18	2.04	1.95	1.87	1.82
	.05	4.00	3.15	2.76	2.53	2.37	2.25	2.17
	.01	7.08	4.98	4.13	3.65	3.34	3.12	2.95
120	.10	2.75	2.35	2.13	1.99	1.90	1.82	1.77
	.05	3.92	3.07	2.68	2.45	2.29	2.17	2.09
	.01	6.85	4.79	3.95	3.48	3.17	2.96	2.79
∞	.10	2.71	2.30	2.08	1.94	1.85	1.77	1.72
	.05	3.84	3.00	2.60	2.37	2.21	2.10	2.01
	.01	6.63	4.61	3.78	3.32	3.02	2.80	2.64

Distribution of F *(continued)*

df denom.	α	df *for Numerator* 8	9	10	12	15	20	24
1	.10	59.44	59.86	60.19	60.71	61.22	61.74	62.00
	.05	238.90	240.50	241.90	243.90	245.90	248.00	249.10
	.01	5981.00	6022.00	6056.00	6106.00	6157.00	6209.00	6235.00
2	.10	9.37	9.38	9.39	9.41	9.42	9.44	9.45
	.05	19.37	19.38	19.40	19.41	19.43	19.45	19.45
	.01	99.37	99.39	99.40	99.42	99.43	99.45	99.46
3	.10	5.25	5.24	5.23	5.22	5.20	5.18	5.18
	.05	8.85	8.81	8.79	8.74	8.70	8.66	8.64
	.01	27.49	27.35	27.23	27.05	26.87	26.69	26.60
4	.10	3.95	3.94	3.92	3.90	3.87	3.84	3.83
	.05	6.04	6.00	5.96	5.91	5.86	5.80	5.77
	.01	14.80	14.66	14.55	14.37	14.20	14.02	13.93
5	.10	3.34	3.32	3.30	3.27	3.24	3.21	3.19
	.05	4.82	4.77	4.74	4.68	4.62	4.56	4.53
	.01	10.29	10.16	10.05	9.89	9.72	9.55	9.47
6	.10	2.98	2.96	2.94	2.90	2.87	2.84	2.82
	.05	4.15	4.10	4.06	4.00	3.94	3.87	3.84
	.01	8.10	7.98	7.87	7.72	7.56	7.40	7.31
7	.10	2.75	2.72	2.70	2.67	2.63	2.59	2.58
	.05	3.73	3.68	3.64	3.57	3.51	3.44	3.41
	.01	6.84	6.72	6.62	6.47	6.31	6.16	6.07
8	.10	2.59	2.56	2.54	2.50	2.46	2.42	2.40
	.05	3.44	3.39	3.35	3.28	3.22	3.15	3.12
	.01	6.03	5.91	5.81	5.67	5.52	5.36	5.28
9	.10	2.47	2.44	2.42	2.38	2.34	2.30	2.28
	.05	3.23	3.18	3.14	3.07	3.01	2.94	2.90
	.01	5.47	5.35	5.26	5.11	4.96	4.81	4.73

Distribution of F *(continued)*

df denom.	α	\multicolumn{7}{c}{df *for Numerator*}						
		8	9	10	12	15	20	24
10	.10	2.38	2.35	2.32	2.28	2.24	2.20	2.18
	.05	3.07	3.02	2.98	2.91	2.85	2.77	2.74
	.01	5.06	4.94	4.85	4.71	4.56	4.41	4.33
11	.10	2.30	2.27	2.25	2.21	2.17	2.12	2.10
	.05	2.95	2.90	2.85	2.79	2.72	2.65	2.61
	.01	4.74	4.63	4.54	4.40	4.25	4.10	4.02
12	.10	2.24	2.21	2.19	2.15	2.10	2.06	2.04
	.05	2.85	2.80	2.75	2.69	2.62	2.54	2.51
	.01	4.50	4.39	4.30	4.16	4.01	3.86	3.78
13	.10	2.20	2.16	2.14	2.10	2.05	2.01	1.98
	.05	2.77	2.71	2.67	2.60	2.53	2.46	2.42
	.01	4.30	4.19	4.10	3.96	3.82	3.66	3.59
14	.10	2.15	2.12	2.10	2.05	2.01	1.96	1.94
	.05	2.70	2.65	2.60	2.53	2.46	2.39	2.35
	.01	4.14	4.03	3.94	3.80	3.66	3.51	3.43
15	.10	2.12	2.09	2.06	2.02	1.97	1.92	1.90
	.05	2.64	2.59	2.54	2.48	2.40	2.33	2.29
	.01	4.00	3.89	3.80	3.67	3.52	3.37	3.29
16	.10	2.09	2.06	2.03	1.99	1.94	1.89	1.87
	.05	2.59	2.54	2.49	2.42	2.35	2.28	2.24
	.01	3.89	3.78	3.69	3.55	3.41	3.26	3.18
17	.10	2.06	2.03	2.00	1.96	1.91	1.86	1.84
	.05	2.55	2.49	2.45	2.38	2.31	2.23	2.19
	.01	3.79	3.68	3.59	3.46	3.31	3.16	3.08
18	.10	2.04	2.00	1.98	1.93	1.89	1.84	1.81
	.05	2.51	2.46	2.41	2.34	2.27	2.19	2.15
	.01	3.71	3.60	3.51	3.37	3.23	3.08	3.00

Distribution of F *(continued)*

df denom.	α	df *for Numerator*						
		8	9	10	12	15	20	24
19	.10	2.02	1.98	1.96	1.91	1.86	1.81	1.79
	.05	2.48	2.42	2.38	2.31	2.23	2.16	2.11
	.01	3.63	3.52	3.43	3.30	3.15	3.00	2.92
20	.10	2.00	1.96	1.94	1.89	1.84	1.79	1.77
	.05	2.45	2.39	2.35	2.28	2.20	2.12	2.08
	.01	3.56	3.46	3.37	3.23	3.09	2.94	2.86
21	.10	1.98	1.95	1.92	1.87	1.83	1.78	1.75
	.05	2.42	2.37	2.32	2.25	2.18	2.10	2.05
	.01	3.51	3.40	3.31	3.17	3.03	2.88	2.80
22	.10	1.97	1.93	1.90	1.86	1.81	1.76	1.73
	.05	2.40	2.34	2.30	2.23	2.15	2.07	2.03
	.01	3.45	3.35	3.26	3.12	2.98	2.83	2.75
23	.10	1.95	1.92	1.89	1.84	1.80	1.74	1.72
	05	2.37	2.32	2.27	2.20	2.13	2.05	2.01
	.01	3.41	3.30	3.21	3.07	2.93	2.78	2.70
24	.10	1.94	1.91	1.88	1.83	1.78	1.73	1.70
	.05	2.36	2.30	2.25	2.18	2.11	2.03	1.98
	.01	3.36	3.26	3.17	3.03	2.89	2.74	2.66
25	.10	1.93	1.89	1.87	1.82	1.77	1.72	1.69
	.05	2.34	2.28	2.24	2.16	2.09	2.01	1.96
	.01	3.32	3.22	3.13	2.99	2.85	2.70	2.62
26	.10	1.92	1.88	1.86	1.81	1.76	1.71	1.68
	.05	2.32	2.27	2.22	2.15	2.07	1.99	1.95
	.01	3.29	3.18	3.09	2.96	2.81	2.66	2.58
27	.10	1.91	1.87	1.85	1.80	1.75	1.70	1.67
	.05	2.31	2.25	2.20	2.13	2.06	1.97	1.93
	.01	3.26	3.15	3.06	2.93	2.78	2.63	2.55

Distribution of F *(continued)*

df denom.	α	8	9	10	12	15	20	24
					df *for Numerator*			
28	.10	1.90	1.87	1.84	1.79	1.74	1.69	1.66
	.05	2.29	2.24	2.19	2.12	2.04	1.96	1.91
	.01	3.23	3.12	3.03	2.90	2.75	2.60	2.52
29	.10	1.89	1.86	1.83	1.78	1.73	1.68	1.65
	.05	2.28	2.22	2.18	2.10	2.03	1.94	1.90
	.01	3.20	3.09	3.00	2.87	2.73	2.57	2.49
30	.10	1.88	1.85	1.82	1.77	1.72	1.67	1.64
	.05	2.27	2.21	2.16	2.09	2.01	1.93	1.89
	.01	3.17	3.07	2.98	2.84	2.70	2.55	2.47
40	.10	1.83	1.79	1.76	1.71	1.66	1.61	1.57
	.05	2.18	2.12	2.08	2.00	1.92	1.84	1.79
	.01	2.99	2.89	2.80	2.66	2.52	2.37	2.29
60	.10	1.77	1.74	1.71	1.66	1.60	1.54	1.51
	.05	2.10	2.04	1.99	1.92	1.84	1.75	1.70
	.01	2.82	2.72	2.63	2.50	2.35	2.20	2.12
120	.10	1.72	1.68	1.65	1.60	1.55	1.48	1.45
	.05	2.02	1.96	1.91	1.83	1.75	1.66	1.61
	.01	2.66	2.56	2.47	2.34	2.19	2.03	1.95
∞	.10	1.67	1.63	1.60	1.55	1.49	1.42	1.38
	.05	1.94	1.88	1.83	1.75	1.67	1.57	1.52
	.01	2.51	2.41	2.32	2.18	2.04	1.88	1.79

Distribution of F *(continued)*

df denom.	α	\multicolumn{5}{c}{df *for Numerator*}
		30	*40*	*60*	*120*	∞
1	.10	62.26	62.53	62.79	63.06	63.33
	.05	250.10	251.10	252.20	253.30	254.30
	.01	6261.00	6287.00	6313.00	6339.00	6366.00
2	.10	9.46	9.47	9.47	9.48	9.49
	.05	19.46	19.47	19.48	19.49	19.50
	.01	99.47	99.47	99.48	99.49	99.50
3	.10	5.17	5.16	5.15	5.14	5.13
	.05	8.62	8.59	8.57	8.55	8.53
	.01	26.50	26.41	26.32	26.22	26.13
4	.10	3.82	3.80	3.79	3.78	3.76
	.05	5.75	5.72	5.69	5.66	5.63
	.01	13.84	13.75	13.65	13.56	13.46
5	.10	3.17	3.16	3.14	3.12	3.10
	.05	4.50	4.46	4.43	4.40	4.36
	.01	9.38	9.29	9.20	9.11	9.02
6	.10	2.80	2.78	2.76	2.74	2.72
	.05	3.81	3.77	3.74	3.70	3.67
	.01	7.23	7.14	7.06	6.97	6.88
7	.10	2.56	2.54	2.51	2.49	2.47
	.05	3.38	3.34	3.30	3.27	3.23
	.01	5.99	5.91	5.82	5.74	5.65
8	.10	2.38	2.36	2.34	2.32	2.29
	.05	3.08	3.04	3.01	2.97	2.93
	.01	5.20	5.12	5.03	4.95	4.86
9	.10	2.25	2.23	2.21	2.18	2.16
	.05	2.86	2.83	2.79	2.75	2.71
	.01	4.65	4.57	4.48	4.40	4.31

Distribution of F *(continued)*

df denom.	α	30	40	60	120	∞
				df *for Numerator*		
10	.10	2.16	2.13	2.11	2.08	2.06
	.05	2.70	2.66	2.62	2.58	2.54
	.01	4.25	4.17	4.08	4.00	3.91
11	.10	2.08	2.05	2.03	2.00	1.97
	.05	2.57	2.53	2.49	2.45	2.40
	.01	3.94	3.86	3.78	3.69	3.60
12	.10	2.01	1.99	1.96	1.93	1.90
	.05	2.47	2.43	2.38	2.34	2.30
	.01	3.70	3.62	3.54	3.45	3.36
13	.10	1.96	1.93	1.90	1.88	1.85
	.05	2.38	2.34	2.30	2.25	2.21
	.01	3.51	3.43	3.34	3.25	3.17
14	.10	1.91	1.89	1.86	1.83	1.80
	.05	2.31	2.27	2.22	2.18	2.13
	.01	3.35	3.27	3.18	3.09	3.00
15	.10	1.87	1.85	1.82	1.79	1.76
	.05	2.25	2.20	2.16	2.11	2.07
	.01	3.21	3.13	3.05	2.96	2.87
16	.10	1.84	1.81	1.78	1.75	1.72
	.05	2.19	2.15	2.11	2.06	2.01
	.01	3.10	3.02	2.93	2.84	2.75
17	.10	1.81	1.78	1.75	1.72	1.69
	.05	2.15	2.10	2.06	2.01	1.96
	.01	3.00	2.92	2.83	2.75	2.65
18	.10	1.78	1.75	1.72	1.69	1.66
	.05	2.11	2.06	2.02	1.97	1.92
	.01	2.92	2.84	2.75	2.66	2.57

Distribution of F *(continued)*

df denom.	α	df *for Numerator* 30	40	60	120	∞
19	.10	1.76	1.73	1.70	1.67	1.63
	.05	2.07	2.03	1.98	1.93	1.88
	.01	2.84	2.76	2.67	2.58	2.49
20	.10	1.74	1.71	1.68	1.64	1.61
	.05	2.04	1.99	1.95	1.90	1.84
	.01	2.78	2.69	2.61	2.52	2.42
21	.10	1.72	1.69	1.66	1.62	1.59
	.05	2.01	1.96	1.92	1.87	1.81
	.01	2.72	2.64	2.55	2.46	2.36
22	.10	1.70	1.67	1.64	1.60	1.57
	.05	1.98	1.94	1.89	1.84	1.78
	.01	2.67	2.58	2.50	2.40	2.31
23	.10	1.69	1.66	1.62	1.59	1.55
	.05	1.96	1.91	1.86	1.81	1.76
	.01	2.62	2.54	2.45	2.35	2.26
24	.10	1.67	1.64	1.61	1.57	1.53
	.05	1.94	1.89	1.84	1.79	1.73
	.01	2.58	2.49	2.40	2.31	2.21
25	.10	1.66	1.63	1.59	1.56	1.52
	.05	1.92	1.87	1.82	1.77	1.71
	.01	2.54	2.45	2.36	2.27	2.17
26	.10	1.65	1.61	1.58	1.54	1.50
	.05	1.90	1.85	1.80	1.75	1.69
	.01	2.50	2.42	2.33	2.23	2.13
27	.10	1.64	1.60	1.57	1.53	1.49
	.05	1.88	1.84	1.79	1.73	1.67
	.01	2.47	2.38	2.29	2.20	2.10

Distribution of F *(continued)*

df denom.		df *for Numerator*				
		30	40	60	120	∞
28	.10	1.63	1.59	1.56	1.52	1.48
	.05	1.87	1.82	1.77	1.71	1.65
	.01	2.44	2.35	2.26	2.17	2.06
29	.10	1.62	1.58	1.55	1.51	1.47
	.05	1.85	1.81	1.75	1.70	1.64
	.01	2.41	2.33	2.23	2.14	2.03
30	.10	1.61	1.57	1.54	1.50	1.46
	.05	1.84	1.79	1.74	1.68	1.62
	.01	2.39	2.30	2.21	2.11	2.01
40	.10	1.54	1.51	1.47	1.42	1.38
	.05	1.74	1.69	1.64	1.58	1.51
	.01	2.20	2.11	2.02	1.92	1.80
60	.10	1.48	1.44	1.40	1.35	1.29
	.05	1.65	1.59	1.53	1.47	1.39
	.01	2.03	1.94	1.84	1.73	1.60
120	.10	1.41	1.37	1.32	1.26	1.19
	.05	1.55	1.50	1.43	1.35	1.25
	.01	1.86	1.76	1.66	1.53	1.38
∞	.10	1.34	1.30	1.24	1.17	1.00
	.05	1.46	1.39	1.32	1.22	1.00
	.01	1.70	1.59	1.47	1.32	1.00

Appendix D

Distribution of χ^2

df	.99	.98	.95	Probability .90	.80	.70	.50	.30
1	.0³157	.0³628	.00393	.0158	.0642	.148	.455	1.074
2	.0201	.0404	.103	.211	.446	.713	1.386	2.408
3	.115	.185	.352	.584	1.005	1.424	2.366	3.665
4	.297	.429	.711	1.064	1.649	2.195	3.357	4.878
5	.554	.752	1.145	1.610	2.343	3.000	4.351	6.064
6	.872	1.134	1.635	2.204	3.070	3.828	5.348	7.231
7	1.239	1.564	2.167	2.833	3.822	4.671	6.346	8.383
8	1.646	2.032	2.733	3.490	4.594	5.527	7.344	9.524
9	2.088	2.532	3.325	4.168	5.380	6.393	8.343	10.656
10	2.558	3.059	3.940	4.865	6.179	7.267	9.342	11.781
11	3.053	3.609	4.575	5.578	6.989	8.148	10.341	12.899
12	3.571	4.178	5.226	6.304	7.807	9.034	11.340	14.011
13	4.107	4.765	5.892	7.042	8.634	9.926	12.340	15.119
14	4.660	5.368	6.571	7.790	9.467	10.821	13.339	16.222
15	5.229	5.985	7.261	8.547	10.307	11.721	14.339	17.322
16	5.812	6.614	7.962	9.312	11.152	12.624	15.338	18.418
17	6.408	7.255	8.672	10.085	12.002	13.531	16.338	19.511
18	7.015	7.906	9.390	10.865	12.857	14.440	17.338	20.601
19	7.633	8.567	10.117	11.651	13.716	15.352	18.338	21.689
20	8.260	9.237	10.851	12.443	14.578	16.266	19.337	22.775
21	8.897	9.915	11.591	13.240	15.445	17.182	20.337	23.858
22	9.542	10.600	12.338	14.041	16.314	18.101	21.337	24.939
23	10.196	11.293	13.091	14.848	17.187	19.021	22.337	26.018
24	10.856	11.992	13.848	15.659	18.062	19.943	23.337	27.096
25	11.524	12.697	14.611	16.473	18.940	20.867	24.337	28.172

Source: From Table IV of R. A. Fisher and F. Yates, *Statistical Tables for Biological, Agricultural and Medical Research*, 6th ed. (London: Longman Group Ltd., 1970), (previously published by Oliver and Boyd, Edinburgh), by permission of the authors and publishers.

Distribution of χ^2 *(continued)*

df	.20	.10	Probability .05	.02	.01	.001
1	1.642	2.706	3.841	5.412	6.635	10.827
2	3.219	4.605	5.991	7.824	9.210	13.815
3	4.642	6.251	7.815	9.837	11.345	16.266
4	5.989	7.779	9.488	11.668	13.277	18.467
5	7.289	9.236	11.070	13.388	15.086	20.515
6	8.558	10.645	12.592	15.033	16.812	22.457
7	9.803	12.017	14.067	16.622	18.475	24.322
8	11.030	13.362	15.507	18.168	20.090	26.125
9	12.242	14.684	16.919	19.679	21.666	27.877
10	13.442	15.987	18.307	21.161	23.209	29.588
11	14.631	17.275	19.675	22.618	24.725	31.264
12	15.812	18.549	21.026	24.054	26.217	32.909
13	16.985	19.812	22.362	25.472	27.688	34.528
14	18.151	21.064	23.685	26.873	29.141	36.123
15	19.311	22.307	24.996	28.259	30.578	37.697
16	20.465	23.542	26.296	29.633	32.000	39.252
17	21.615	24.769	27.587	30.995	33.409	40.790
18	22.760	25.989	28.869	32.346	34.805	42.312
19	23.900	27.204	30.144	33.687	36.191	43.820
20	25.038	28.412	31.410	35.020	37.566	45.315
21	26.171	29.615	32.671	36.343	38.932	46.797
22	27.301	30.813	33.924	37.659	40.289	48.268
23	28.429	32.007	35.172	38.968	41.638	49.728
24	29.553	33.196	36.415	40.270	42.980	51.179
25	30.675	34.382	37.652	41.566	44.314	52.620

Distribution of χ^2 *(*continued*)*

df	.99	.98	.95	Probability .90	.80	.70	.50	.30
26	12.198	13.409	15.379	17.292	19.820	21.792	25.336	29.246
27	12.879	14.125	16.151	18.114	20.703	22.719	26.336	30.319
28	13.565	14.847	16.928	18.939	21.588	23.647	27.336	31.391
29	14.256	15.574	17.708	19.768	22.475	24.577	28.336	32.461
30	14.953	16.306	18.493	20.599	23.364	25.508	29.336	33.530
32	16.362	17.783	20.072	22.271	25.148	27.373	31.336	35.665
34	17.789	19.275	21.664	23.952	26.938	29.242	33.336	37.795
36	19.233	20.783	23.269	25.643	28.735	31.115	35.336	39.922
38	20.691	22.304	24.884	27.343	30.537	32.992	37.335	42.045
40	22.164	23.838	26.509	29.051	32.345	34.872	39.335	44.165
42	23.650	25.383	28.144	30.765	34.157	36.755	41.335	46.282
44	25.148	26.939	29.787	32.487	35.974	38.641	43.335	48.396
46	26.657	28.504	31.439	34.215	37.795	40.529	45.335	50.507
48	28.177	30.080	33.098	35.949	39.621	42.420	47.335	52.616
50	29.707	31.664	34.764	37.689	41.449	44.313	49.335	54.723
52	31.246	33.256	36.437	39.433	43.281	46.209	51.335	56.827
54	32.793	34.856	38.116	41.183	45.117	48.106	53.335	58.930
56	34.350	36.464	39.801	42.937	46.955	50.005	55.335	61.031
58	35.913	38.078	41.492	44.696	48.797	51.906	57.335	63.129
60	37.485	39.699	43.188	46.459	50.641	53.809	59.335	65.227
62	39.063	41.327	44.889	48.226	52.487	55.714	61.335	67.322
64	40.649	42.960	46.595	49.996	54.336	57.620	63.335	69.416
66	42.240	44.599	48.305	51.770	56.188	59.527	65.335	71.508
68	43.848	46.244	50.020	53.548	58.042	61.436	67.335	73.600
70	45.442	47.893	51.739	55.329	59.898	63.346	69.334	75.689

Distribution of χ^2 *(continued)*

df	.20	.10	Probability .05	.02	.01	.001
26	31.795	35.563	38.885	42.856	45.642	54.052
27	32.912	36.741	40.113	44.140	46.963	55.476
28	34.027	37.916	41.337	45.419	48.278	56.893
29	35.139	39.087	42.557	46.693	49.588	58.302
30	36.250	40.256	43.773	47.962	50.892	59.703
32	38.466	42.585	46.194	50.487	53.486	62.487
34	40.676	44.903	48.602	52.995	56.061	65.247
36	42.879	47.212	50.999	55.489	58.619	67.985
38	45.076	49.513	53.384	57.969	61.162	70.703
40	47.269	51.805	55.759	60.436	63.691	73.402
42	49.456	54.090	58.124	62.892	66.206	76.084
44	51.639	56.369	60.481	65.337	68.710	78.750
46	53.818	58.641	62.830	67.771	71.201	81.400
48	55.993	60.907	65.171	70.197	73.683	84.037
50	58.164	63.167	67.505	72.613	76.154	86.661
52	60.332	65.422	69.832	75.021	78.616	89.272
54	62.496	67.673	72.153	77.422	81.069	91.872
56	64.658	69.919	74.468	79.815	83.513	94.461
58	66.816	72.160	76.778	82.201	85.950	97.039
60	68.972	74.397	79.082	84.580	88.379	99.607
62	71.125	76.630	81.381	86.953	90.802	102.166
64	73.276	78.860	83.675	89.320	93.217	104.716
66	75.424	81.085	85.965	91.681	95.626	107.258
68	77.571	83.308	88.250	94.037	98.028	109.791
70	79.715	85.527	90.531	96.388	100.425	112.317

Appendix E

Table of critical values of U

						Two-tailed test at $\alpha = .05$						
n_1	n_2	9	10	11	12	13	14	15	16	17	18	19	20
	1												
	2	0	0	0	1	1	1	1	1	2	2	2	2
	3	2	3	3	4	4	5	5	6	6	7	7	8
	4	4	5	6	7	8	9	10	11	11	12	13	13
	5	7	8	9	11	12	13	14	15	17	18	19	20
	6	10	11	13	14	16	17	19	21	22	24	25	27
	7	12	14	16	18	20	22	24	26	28	30	32	34
	8	15	17	19	22	24	26	29	31	34	36	38	41
	9	17	20	23	26	28	31	34	37	39	42	45	48
	10	20	23	26	29	33	36	39	42	45	48	52	55
	11	23	26	30	33	37	40	44	47	51	55	58	62
	12	26	29	33	37	41	45	49	53	57	61	65	69
	13	28	33	37	41	45	50	54	59	63	67	72	76
	14	31	36	40	45	50	55	59	64	67	74	78	83
	15	34	39	44	49	54	59	64	70	75	80	85	90
	16	37	42	47	53	59	64	70	75	81	86	92	98
	17	39	45	51	57	63	67	75	81	87	93	99	105
	18	42	48	55	61	67	74	80	86	93	99	106	112
	19	45	52	58	65	72	78	85	92	99	106	113	119
	20	48	55	62	69	76	83	90	98	105	112	119	127

Source: From Tables 2 and 5 of D. Auble, "Extended tables for the Mann-Whitney statistic," *Bulletin of the Institute of Educational Research at Indiana University,* 1953, 1:15–30, by permission of the Institute of Educational Research.

Table of critical values of U *(continued)*

							Two-tailed test at $\alpha = .01$					
n_1	n_2	9	10	11	12	13	14	15	16	17	18	19	20
	1												
	2											0	0
	3	0	0	0	1	1	1	2	2	2	2	3	3
	4	1	2	2	3	3	4	5	5	6	6	7	8
	5	3	4	5	6	7	7	8	9	10	11	12	13
	6	5	6	7	9	10	11	12	13	15	16	17	18
	7	7	9	10	12	13	15	16	18	19	21	22	24
	8	9	11	13	15	17	18	20	22	24	26	28	30
	9	11	13	16	18	20	22	24	27	29	31	33	36
	10	13	16	18	21	24	26	29	31	34	37	39	42
	11	16	18	21	24	27	30	33	36	39	42	45	48
	12	18	21	24	27	31	34	37	41	44	47	51	54
	13	20	24	27	31	34	38	42	45	49	53	56	60
	14	22	26	30	34	38	42	46	50	54	58	63	67
	15	24	29	33	37	42	46	51	55	60	64	69	73
	16	27	31	36	41	45	50	55	60	65	70	74	79
	17	29	34	39	44	49	54	60	65	70	75	81	86
	18	31	37	42	47	53	58	64	70	75	81	87	92
	19	33	39	45	51	56	63	69	74	81	87	93	99
	20	36	42	48	54	60	67	73	79	86	92	99	105

Appendix F

Probability of obtaining a U *not larger than that tabulated in comparing samples of size* n_1 *and* n_2

	$n_2 = 3$		
U \ n_1	1	2	3
0	.250	.100	.050
1	.500	.200	.100
2	.750	.400	.200
3		.600	.350
4			.500
5			.650

	$n_2 = 4$			
U \ n_1	1	2	3	4
0	.200	.067	.028	.014
1	.400	.133	.057	.029
2	.600	.267	.114	.057
3		.400	.200	.100
4		.600	.314	.171
5			.429	.243
6			.571	.343
7				.443
8				.557

Source: From Table I of H. B. Mann and D. R. Whitney, "On a test of whether one of two random variables is stochastically larger than the other," *Annals of Mathematical Statistics,* 1947, 18:52–54, by permission of the Institute of Mathematical Statistics.

Probability of obtaining a U not larger than that tabulated in comparing samples of size n_1 and n_2 (continued)

			$n_2 = 5$		
U \ n_1	1	2	3	4	5
0	.167	.047	.018	.008	.004
1	.333	.095	.036	.016	.008
2	.500	.190	.071	.032	.016
3	.667	.286	.125	.056	.028
4		.429	.196	.095	.048
5		.571	.286	.143	.075
6			.393	.206	.111
7			.500	.278	.155
8			.607	.365	.210
9				.452	.274
10				.548	.345
11					.421
12					.500
13					.579

			$n_2 = 6$			
U \ n_1	1	2	3	4	5	6
0	.143	.036	.012	.005	.002	.001
1	.286	.071	.024	.010	.004	.002
2	.428	.143	.048	.019	.009	.004
3	.571	.214	.083	.033	.015	.008
4		.321	.131	.057	.026	.013
5		.429	.190	.086	.041	.021
6		.571	.274	.129	.063	.032
7			.357	.176	.089	.047
8			.452	.238	.123	.066
9			.548	.305	.165	.090
10				.381	.214	.120
11				.457	.268	.155
12				.545	.331	.197
13					.396	.242
14					.465	.294
15					.535	.350
16						.409
17						.469
18						.531

Probability of obtaining a U *not larger than that tabulated in comparing samples of size* n_1 *and* n_2 *(continued)*

U \ n_1	1	2	3	4	5	6	7
				$n_2 = 7$			
0	.125	.028	.008	.003	.001	.001	.000
1	.250	.056	.017	.006	.003	.001	.001
2	.375	.111	.033	.012	.005	.002	.001
3	.500	.167	.058	.021	.009	.004	.002
4	.625	.250	.092	.036	.015	.007	.003
5		.333	.133	.055	.024	.011	.006
6		.444	.192	.082	.037	.017	.009
7		.556	.258	.115	.053	.026	.013
8			.333	.158	.074	.037	.019
9			.417	.206	.101	.051	.027
10			.500	.264	.134	.069	.036
11			.583	.324	.172	.090	.049
12				.394	.216	.117	.064
13				.464	.265	.147	.082
14				.538	.319	.183	.104
15					.378	.223	.130
16					.438	.267	.159
17					.500	.314	.191
18					.562	.365	.228
19						.418	.267
20						.473	.310
21						.527	.355
22							.402
23							.451
24							.500
25							.549

Probability of obtaining a U *not larger than that tabulated in comparing samples of size* n_1 *and* n_2

				$n_2 = 8$				
U \ n_1	*1*	*2*	*3*	*4*	*5*	*6*	*7*	*8*
0	.111	.022	.006	.002	.001	.000	.000	.000
1	.222	.044	.012	.004	.002	.001	.000	.000
2	.333	.089	.024	.008	.003	.001	.001	.000
3	.444	.133	.042	.014	.005	.002	.001	.001
4	.556	.200	.067	.024	.009	.004	.002	.001
5		.267	.097	.036	.015	.006	.003	.001
6		.356	.139	.055	.023	.010	.005	.002
7		.444	.188	.077	.033	.015	.007	.003
8		.556	.248	.107	.047	.021	.010	.005
9			.315	.141	.064	.030	.014	.007
10			.387	.184	.085	.041	.020	.010
11			.461	.230	.111	.054	.027	.014
12			.539	.285	.142	.071	.036	.019
13				.341	.177	.091	.047	.025
14				.404	.217	.114	.060	.032
15				.467	.262	.141	.076	.041
16				.533	.311	.172	.095	.052
17					.362	.207	.116	.065
18					.416	.245	.140	.080
19					.472	.286	.168	.097
20					.528	.331	.198	.117
21						.377	.232	.139
22						.426	.268	.164
23						.475	.306	.191
24						.525	.347	.221
25							.389	.253
26							.433	.287
27							.478	.323
28							.522	.360
29								.399
30								.439
31								.480
32								.520

Appendix G

Table of critical values for the Wilcoxon test

N	.05 .10	.025 .05	.01 .02	.005 P *one-tailed* .01 P *two-tailed*
5	1			
6	2	1		
7	4	2	0	
8	6	4	2	0
9	8	6	3	2
10	11	8	5	3
11	14	11	7	5
12	17	14	10	7
13	21	17	13	10
14	26	21	16	13
15	30	25	20	16
16	36	30	24	19
17	41	35	28	23
18	47	40	33	28
19	54	46	38	32
20	60	52	43	37
21	68	59	49	43
22	75	66	56	49
23	83	73	62	55
24	92	81	69	61
25	101	90	77	68

Source: From Table 2 of F. Wilcoxon, and R. A. Wilcoxon, *Some rapid approximate statistical procedures* (Pearl River, N.Y.: Lederle Laboratories, a Division of American Cyanamid Company, 1964), by permission of Lederle Laboratories.

Appendix H

Transformation of r *to* z′

z′	.00	.01	.02	.03	.04	.05	.06	.07	.08	.09
.0	.0000	.0100	.0200	.0300	.0400	.0500	.0599	.0699	.0798	.0898
.1	.0997	.1096	.1194	.1293	.1391	.1489	.1586	.1684	.1781	.1877
.2	.1974	.2070	.2165	.2260	.2355	.2449	.2543	.2636	.2729	.2821
.3	.2913	.3004	.3095	.3185	.3275	.3364	.3452	.3540	.3627	.3714
.4	.3800	.3885	.3969	.4053	.4136	.4219	.4301	.4382	.4462	.4542
.5	.4621	.4699	.4777	.4854	.4930	.5005	.5080	.5154	.5227	.5299
.6	.5370	.5441	.5511	.5580	.5649	.5717	.5784	.5850	.5915	.5980
.7	.6044	.6107	.6169	.6231	.6291	.6351	.6411	.6469	.6527	.6584
.8	.6640	.6696	.6751	.6805	.6858	.6911	.6963	.7014	.7064	.7114
.9	.7163	.7211	.7259	.7306	.7352	.7398	.7443	.7487	.7531	.7574
1.0	.7616	.7658	.7699	.7739	.7779	.7818	.7857	.7895	.7932	.7969
1.1	.8005	.8041	.8076	.8110	.8144	.8178	.8210	.8243	.8275	.8306
1.2	.8337	.8367	.8397	.8426	.8455	.8483	.8511	.8538	.8565	.8591
1.3	.8617	.8643	.8668	.8692	.8717	.8741	.8764	.8787	.8810	.8832
1.4	.8854	.8875	.8896	.8917	.8937	.8957	.8977	.8996	.9015	.9033
1.5	.9051	.9069	.9087	.9104	.9121	.9138	.9154	.9170	.9186	.9201
1.6	.9217	.9232	.9246	.9261	.9275	.9289	.9302	.9316	.9329	.9341
1.7	.9354	.9366	.9379	.9391	.9402	.9414	.9425	.9436	.9447	.9458
1.8	.9468	.9478	.9488	.9498	.9508	.9518	.9527	.9536	.9545	.9554
1.9	.9562	.9571	.9579	.9587	.9595	.9603	.9611	.9619	.9626	.9633
2.0	.9640	.9647	.9654	.9661	.9668	.9674	.9680	.9687	.9693	.9699
2.1	.9705	.9710	.9716	.9722	.9727	.9732	.9738	.9743	.9748	.9753
2.2	.9757	.9762	.9767	.9771	.9776	.9780	.9785	.9789	.9793	.9797
2.3	.9801	.9805	.9809	.9812	.9816	.9820	.9823	.9827	.9830	.9834
2.4	.9837	.9840	.9843	.9846	.9849	.9852	.9855	.9858	.9861	.9864
2.5	.9866	.9869	.9871	.9874	.9876	.9879	.9881	.9884	.9886	.9888
2.6	.9890	.9892	.9895	.9897	.9899	.9901	.9903	.9905	.9906	.9908
2.7	.9910	.9912	.9914	.9915	.9917	.9919	.9920	.9922	.9923	.9925
2.8	.9926	.9928	.9929	.9931	.9932	.9933	.9935	.9936	.9937	.9938
2.9	.9940	.9941	.9942	.9943	.9944	.9945	.9946	.9948	.9949	.9950
3.0	.9951									
3.1	.9960									
3.2	.9967									
3.3	.9973									
3.4	.9978									
3.5	.9982									

Source: From Table VII of R. A. Fisher and F. Yates, *Statistical Tables for Biological, Agricultural and Medical Research*, 6th ed. (London: Longman Group Ltd., 1970), (previously published by Oliver and Boyd, Edinburgh), by permission of the authors and publishers.

Transformation of r *to* z' *(*continued*)*

z'	.00	.01	.02	.03	.04	.05	.06	.07	.08	.09
3.6	.9985									
3.7	.9988									
3.8	.9990									
3.9	.9992									
4.0	.9993									
4.1	.9995									
4.2	.9996									
4.3	.9996									
4.4	.9997									
4.5	.9998									

Appendix I

Table of probabilities associated with values as large as observed values of H
in the Kruskal-Wallis test

n₁	n₂	n₃	H	Probability	n₁	n₂	n₃	H	Probability
Sample sizes					Sample sizes				
2	1	1	2.7000	.500	4	1	1	3.5714	.200
2	2	1	3.6000	.267					
					4	2	1	4.8214	.057
2	2	2	4.5714	.067				4.5000	.076
			3.7143	.200				4.0179	.114
3	1	1	3.2000	.300	4	2	2	6.0000	.014
								5.3333	.033
3	2	1	4.2857	.100				5.1250	.052
			3.8571	.133				4.3750	.100
								4.1667	.105
3	2	2	5.3572	.029					
			4.7143	.048	4	3	1	5.8333	.021
			4.5000	.067				5.2083	.050
			4.4643	.105				5.0000	.057
								4.0556	.093
3	3	1	5.1429	.043				3.8889	.129
			4.5714	.100					
			4.0000	.129	4	3	2	6.4444	.009
								6.4222	.010
3	3	2	6.2500	.011				5.4444	.047
			5.3611	.032				5.4000	.052
			5.1389	.061				4.5111	.098
			4.5556	.100				4.4667	.101
			4.2500	.121					
					4	3	3	6.7455	.010
3	3	3	7.2000	.004				6.7091	.013
			6.4889	.001				5.7909	.046
			5.6889	.029				5.7273	.050
			5.6000	.050				4.7091	.094
			5.0667	.086				4.7000	.101
			4.6222	.100					

Source: From Table 6.1 of W. H. Kruskal and W. A. Wallis, "Use of ranks in one-criterion variance analyses," *Journal of the American Statistical Association,* 1952, 47:614–617, by permission of the American Statistical Association.

Table of probabilities associated with values as large as observed values of H *in the Kruskal-Wallis test (continued)*

n_1	n_2	n_3	H	Probability	n_1	n_2	n_3	H	Probability
4	4	1	6.6667	.010	5	2	2	6.5333	.008
			6.1667	.022				6.1333	.013
			4.9667	.048				5.1600	.034
			4.8667	.054				5.0400	.056
			4.1667	.082				4.3733	.090
			4.0667	.102				4.2933	.122
4	4	2	7.0364	.006	5	3	1	6.4000	.012
			6.8727	.011				4.9600	.048
			5.4545	.046				4.8711	.052
			5.2364	.052				4.0178	.095
			4.5545	.098				3.8400	.123
			4.4455	.103					
					5	3	2	6.9091	.009
4	4	3	7.1439	.010				6.8218	.010
			7.1364	.011				5.2509	.049
			5.5985	.049				5.1055	.052
			5.5758	.051				4.6509	.091
			4.5455	.099				4.4945	.101
			4.4773	.102					
					5	3	3	6.9818	.010
4	4	4	7.6538	.008				6.8606	.011
			7.5385	.011				5.4424	.048
			5.6923	.049				5.3455	.050
			5.6538	.054				4.5333	.097
			4.6539	.097				4.4121	.109
			4.5001	.104					
					5	4	1	6.9545	.008
5	1	1	3.8571	.143				6.8400	.011
								4.9855	.044
5	2	1	5.2500	.036				4.8600	.056
			5.0000	.048				3.9873	.098
			4.4500	.071				3.9600	.102
			4.2000	.095					
			4.0500	.119					

Table of probabilities associated with values as large as observed values of H
*in the Kruskal-Wallis test (*continued*)*

Sample sizes					Sample Sizes				
n_1	n_2	n_3	H	Probability	n_1	n_2	n_3	H	Probability
5	4	2	7.2045	.009	5	5	2	7.3385	.010
			7.1182	.010				7.2692	.010
			5.2727	.049				5.3385	.047
			5.2682	.050				5.2462	.051
			4.5409	.098				4.6231	.097
			4.5182	.101				4.5077	.100
5	4	3	7.4449	.010	5	5	3	7.5780	.010
			7.3949	.011				7.5429	.010
			5.6564	.049				5.7055	.046
			5.6308	.050				5.6264	.051
			4.5487	.099				4.5451	.100
			4.5231	.103				4.5363	.102
5	4	4	7.7604	.009	5	5	4	7.8229	.010
			7.7440	.011				7.7914	.010
			5.6571	.049				5.6657	.049
			5.6176	.050				5.6429	.050
			4.6187	.100				4.5229	.099
			4.5527	.102				4.5200	.101
5	5	1	7.3091	.009	5	5	5	8.0000	.009
			6.8364	.011				7.9800	.010
			5.1273	.046				5.7800	.049
			4.9091	.053				5.6600	.051
			4.1091	.086				4.5600	.100
			4.0364	.105				4.5000	.102

Appendix J

Exact distribution of Friedman test for n from 2 to 9, three sets of ranks, and for n from 2 to 4, four sets of ranks

χ_r^2	$k = 3;\ n = 2$ P	χ_r^2	$k = 3;\ n = 3$ P	χ_r^2	$k = 3;\ n = 4$ P
0	1.000	0.000	1.000	0.0	1.000
1	.833	0.667	.944	0.5	.931
3	.500	2.000	.528	1.5	.653
4	.167	2.667	.361	2.0	.431
		4.667	.194	3.5	.273
		6.000	.028	4.5	.125
				6.0	.069
				6.5	.042
				8.0	.0046

χ_r^2	$k = 3;\ n = 5$ P	χ_r^2	$k = 3;\ n = 6$ P	χ_r^2	$k = 3;\ n = 7$ P
0.0	1.000	0.00	1.000	0.000	1.000
0.4	.954	0.33	.956	0.286	.964
1.2	.691	1.00	.740	0.857	.768
1.6	.522	1.33	.570	1.143	.620
2.8	.367	2.33	.430	2.000	.486
3.6	.182	3.00	.252	2.571	.305
4.8	.124	4.00	.184	3.429	.237
5.2	.093	4.33	.142	3.714	.192
6.4	.039	5.33	.072	4.571	.112
7.6	.024	6.33	.052	5.429	.085
8.4	.0085	7.00	.029	6.000	.052
10.0	.00077	8.33	.012	7.143	.027
		9.00	.0081	7.714	.021
		9.33	.0055	8.000	.016
		10.33	.0017	8.857	.0084
		12.00	.00013	10.286	.0036
				10.571	.0027
				11.143	.0012
				12.286	.00032
				14.000	.000021

Source: From Tables V and VI of M. Friedman: "The use of ranks to avoid the assumptions of normality implicit in the analysis of variance," *Journal of the American Statistical Association*, 1937, 32:688–689, by permission of the American Statistical Association.

Exact distribution of Friedman test for n *from 2 to 9, three sets of ranks, and for* n *from 2 to 4, four sets of ranks* (continued)

χ_r^2	P	χ_r^2	P
k=3; n=8		k=3; n=9	
0.00	1.000	0.000	1.000
0.25	.967	0.222	.971
0.75	.794	0.667	.814
1.00	.654	0.889	.865
1.75	.531	1.556	.569
2.25	.355	2.000	.398
3.00	.285	2.667	.328
3.25	.236	2.889	.278
4.00	.149	3.556	.187
4.75	.120	4.222	.154
5.25	.079	4.667	.107
6.25	.047	5.556	.069
6.75	.038	6.000	.057
7.00	.030	6.222	.048
7.75	.018	6.889	.031
9.00	.0099	8.000	.019
9.25	.0080	8.222	.016
9.75	.0048	8.667	.010
10.75	.0024	9.556	.0060
12.00	.0011	10.667	.0035
12.25	.00086	10.889	.0029
13.00	.00026	11.556	.0013
14.25	.000061	12.667	.00066
16.00	.0000036	13.556	.00035
		14.000	.00020
		14.222	.000097
		14.889	.000054
		16.222	.000011
		18.000	.0000006

*Exact distribution of Friedman test for n from 2 to 9, three sets of ranks,
and for n from 2 to 4, four sets of ranks* (continued)

χ_r^2	k = 4; n = 2 P	χ_r^2	k = 4; n = 3 P
0.0	1.000	0.2	1.000
0.6	.958	0.6	.958
1.2	.834	1.0	.910
1.8	.792	1.8	.727
2.4	.625	2.2	.608
3.0	.542	2.6	.524
3.6	.458	3.4	.446
4.2	.375	3.8	.342
4.8	.208	4.2	.300
5.4	.167	5.0	.207
6.0	.042	5.4	.175
		5.8	.148
		6.6	.075
		7.0	.054
		7.4	.033
		8.2	.017
		9.0	.0017

χ_r^2	k = 4; n = 4 P	χ_r^2	k = 4; n = 4 P
0.0	1.000	5.7	.141
0.3	.992	6.0	.105
0.6	.928	6.3	.094
0.9	.900	6.6	.077
1.2	.800	6.9	.068
1.5	.754	7.2	.054
1.8	.677	7.5	.052
2.1	.649	7.8	.036
2.4	.524	8.1	.033
2.7	.508	8.4	.019
3.0	.432	8.7	.014
3.3	.389	9.3	.012
3.6	.355	9.6	.0069
3.9	.324	9.9	.0062
4.5	.242	10.2	.0027
4.8	.200	10.8	.0016
5.1	.190	11.1	.00094
5.4	.158	12.0	.000072

Bibliography

Edwards, A. L. *Statistical methods,* 2nd ed. (New York: Holt, Rinehart & Winston, 1967).

Fisher, R. A. and F. Yates. *Statistical tables for biological, agricultural and medical research,* 6th ed. (Darien, Conn.: Hafner Publishing Co., 1970).

Pearson, E. S. and H. O. Hartley. *Biometrika tables for statisticians,* Vol. I, 3rd ed. (Cambridge: Cambridge University Press, 1970).

Pirie, W. R. and M. A. Hamdan, "Some revised continuity corrections for discrete distributions," *Biometrics,* 1972, 28:693–701.

Siegel, S. *Nonparametric statistics* (New York: McGraw-Hill, 1956).

Winer, B. J. *Statistical principles in experimental design,* 2nd ed. (New York: McGraw-Hill, 1971).

Answers to Exercises

Answers to Exercises

Exercise 2

1. 50 to 1
2. 0.0196
3. 4.4/1000

Exercise 3

$Mo = 3$
$Md = 4$
$\overline{X} = 4.4$

Exercise 4

range $= 8$
$Q = 1$
$s = 1.99$

Exercise 5

$r = 0.81$

Exercise 6

$\hat{Y} = 1.87 + 4.76X$
$\hat{X} = 2.44 + .14Y$
$s_{yx} = 11.15$
$s_{xy} = 1.90$

Exercise 7

1. $\eta_{yx} = 0.998$
2. $\phi = 0.04$
3. $\rho = 0.75$

Exercise 10

1. $t = 3.26$, $df = 28$, $P \leq .01$
2. $t = 1.13$, $df = 9$, not significant
3. $X = 75.4$, $\beta = .59$, power $= .41$

Exercise 11

1. $P \leq .001$
2. $P \leq .001$
3. $t = 1.97$, not significant
4. $\chi^2 = 4.41$, $P \leq .05$
5. $z = 1.47$, not significant

Exercise 12

1.

Source	SS	df	MS	F
Total	555	17		
Between	417	2	208.50	22.66*
Within	138	15	9.20	

$F_{1-2} = 27.57^{**}$ $F_{1-3} = 1.05$ $F_{2-3} = 39.41^{**}$

2.

Source	SS	df	MS	F
Total	2100	39		
Between subjects	1447	9		
Within subjects	653	30		
Treatments	348	3	116.00	10.27**
Error	305	27	11.30	

Exercise 13

1. $\chi^2 = 4.87$, $df = 1$, $P \leq .05$
2. $\chi^2 = 121.31$, $df = 3$, $P \leq .001$

Exercise 14

1. (a) $z = 2.86$, $P \leq .01$
   (b) $P \leq .02$
2. $U_1 = 28.5$, $P \leq .05$
3. $H = 11.66$, $P \leq .01$
4. $\chi_r^2 = 13.62$, $P \leq .01$

Index

Index